T0172496

THE TRAUMA RECOVERY GROUP

The
TRAUMA RECOVERY
GROUP

A GUIDE FOR PRACTITIONERS

Michaela Mendelsohn
Judith Lewis Herman
Emily Schatzow
Melissa Coco
Diya Kallivayalil
Jocelyn Levitan

THE GUILFORD PRESS
New York   London

© 2011 The Guilford Press
A Division of Guilford Publications, Inc.
72 Spring Street, New York, NY 10012
www.guilford.com

All rights reserved

Except as indicated, no part of this book may be reproduced, translated, stored in a retrieval system, or
transmitted, in any form or by any means, electronic, mechanical, photocopying, microfilming, recording, or otherwise, without written permission from the publisher.

Printed in the United States of America

This book is printed on acid-free paper.

Last digit is print number: 9   8   7   6   5   4

LIMITED PHOTOCOPY LICENSE

These materials are intended for use only by qualified professionals.

The publisher grants to individual purchasers of this book nonassignable permission to reproduce
all materials for which photocopying permission is specifically granted in a footnote. This license
is limited to you, the individual purchaser, for personal use or use with individual clients. This
license does not grant the right to reproduce these materials for resale, redistribution, electronic
display, or any other purposes (including but not limited to books, pamphlets, articles, video- or
audiotapes, blogs, file-sharing sites, Internet or intranet sites, and handouts or slides for lectures,
workshops, webinars, or therapy groups, whether or not a fee is charged). Permission to reproduce
these materials for these and any other purposes must be obtained in writing from the Permissions
Department of Guilford Publications.

The authors have checked with sources believed to be reliable in their efforts to provide information
that is complete and generally in accord with the standards of practice that are accepted at the time of
publication. However, in view of the possibility of human error or changes in behavioral, mental health,
or medical sciences, neither the authors, nor the editor and publisher, nor any other party who has been
involved in the preparation or publication of this work warrants that the information contained herein
is in every respect accurate or complete, and they are not responsible for any errors or omissions or the
results obtained from the use of such information. Readers are encouraged to confirm the information
contained in this book with other sources.

Library of Congress Cataloging-in-Publication Data

Mendelsohn, Michaela, 1970– author.
   The trauma recovery group : a guide for practitioners / by Michaela Mendelsohn, Judith Lewis
Herman, Emily Schatzow, Melissa Coco, Diya Kallivayalil, and Jocelyn Levitan.
      p. ; cm.
   Includes bibliographical references and index.
   ISBN 978-1-60918-057-7 (pbk.: alk. paper)
   1. Post-traumatic stress disorder—Treatment.   I. Herman, Judith Lewis, 1942– author.
II. Schatzow, Emily, author.   III. Coco, Melissa, author.   IV. Kallivayalil, Diya, author.   V. Levitan,
Jocelyn, author.   VI. Title.
   [DNLM: 1. Stress Disorders, Post-Traumatic—therapy.   2. Psychotherapy,   Group—methods.
3. Sex Offenses—psychology.   4. Survivors—psychology.   5. Violence—psychology.   WM 172]
   RC552.P67M454 2011
   616.85′210651—dc22
                                                                                        2010050020

About the Authors

Michaela Mendelsohn, PhD, is a psychologist in private practice in Cambridge and Wellesley, Massachusetts, with a specialty in the treatment of trauma-related disorders. She is also a faculty member in the Department of Psychiatry at Harvard Medical School. Dr. Mendelsohn completed a postdoctoral fellowship in the assessment and treatment of trauma survivors at the Victims of Violence (VOV) Program at the Cambridge Health Alliance (CHA), where she subsequently worked as a clinician and researcher and continues to provide supervision and consultation. She also completed postgraduate training in group psychotherapy at the Northeastern Society for Group Psychotherapy. She has published works on a variety of topics related to psychological trauma, including the impact of political violence on youth, interventions for sexually abused children, profiling and school violence, gender and the experience of trauma, and group psychotherapy for trauma survivors.

Judith Lewis Herman, MD, is Clinical Professor of Psychiatry at Harvard Medical School and Director of Training at the VOV Program at the CHA. She is the author of two award-winning books, *Father–Daughter Incest* and *Trauma and Recovery*. Dr. Herman has lectured widely on the subject of sexual and domestic violence. She is the recipient of the 1996 Lifetime Achievement Award from the International Society for Traumatic Stress Studies and the 2000 Woman in Science Award from the American Medical Women's Association. In 2007, Dr. Herman was named a Distinguished Life Fellow of the American Psychiatric Association.

Emily Schatzow, MEd, is a psychotherapist in private practice in Cambridge, Massachusetts, and a trainer and senior consultant for VISIONS, Inc., a nonprofit organization advising public and private institutions on workplace diversity. As a Lecturer in Psychiatry at Harvard Medical School, she was centrally involved in the continuing education conference series, "Learning from Women: Theory and Practice," which has enrolled almost 10,000 participants since 1987. Ms. Schatzow recently held an adjunct faculty appointment at Episcopal Divinity School in Cambridge. She served as the coordinator of group services for the VOV program at the CHA for more than a decade, and during this time she developed and supervised several novel groups for survivors of complex trauma. She is now a Research Associate in Psychiatry at the VOV Program at the CHA/Harvard Medical School. She conducts ongoing consultation groups for clinicians with Dr. Herman in her private practice and has provided extensive teaching and supervision on trauma-related topics.

Melissa Coco, LICSW, is a senior clinician and supervisor at the VOV Program and the Outpatient Psychiatry Department at the CHA, where she is also centrally involved in social work graduate training. She is a faculty member in the Department of Psychiatry at Harvard Medical School. She has completed extensive postgraduate training in the treatment of complex trauma at the VOV Program as well as in psychodynamic psychotherapy at the Program for Psychotherapy at the CHA. Ms. Coco has co-lead and supervised the Trauma Recovery Group for the past 15 years. She has lectured on topics related to the treatment of complex trauma, including group psychotherapy with trauma survivors.

Diya Kallivayalil, PhD, is a staff psychologist in the Outpatient Psychiatry Department at the CHA and a faculty member in the Department of Psychiatry at Harvard Medical School. She completed a 2-year postdoctoral fellowship at the VOV Program, specializing in the assessment and treatment of psychological trauma. In addition to her clinical practice, Dr. Kallivayalil has published in the areas of psychological trauma, feminist therapy, the impact of trauma and migration on mental health in minority and immigrant communities, narrative methods, and cultural and gender socialization and identity in minority communities.

Jocelyn Levitan, MA, is a doctoral student in the Counseling, Clinical and School Psychology Program at the University of California, Santa Barbara. After completing her undergraduate studies, she worked for 2 years as Research Coordinator for multiple grant-funded projects at the VOV Program at the CHA. In her doctoral studies, Ms. Levitan has been involved in quantitative and qualitative research related to interventions for children and adolescents who have been abused and to the expression of trauma and resilience in refugee and immigrant populations. She is currently investigating the therapeutic factors involved in a group therapy program for Latino children who have experienced domestic violence and is completing her clinical practicum at the Child Abuse Listening and Mediation Center (CALM) in Santa Barbara, where she conducts therapy and assessment with children and families who have experienced trauma.

Preface

The Trauma Recovery Group (TRG) had its origins during the late 1970s, as part of a feminist project to revise the understanding of women's psychology and to raise public awareness of the impact of gender-based violence. Judith Lewis Herman and a colleague, Lisa Hirschman, had recently published an interview study of survivors of father–daughter incest (Herman & Hirschman, 1977). The response to this paper indicated that incest was indeed much more common than had been previously recognized. It seemed important, therefore, to devise an effective treatment for incest survivors, one that would address the issues of shame and secrecy that had effectively silenced and isolated so many survivors.

In 1978, Judith Herman and Emily Schatzow visited treatment programs in the United States that worked with victims of childhood sexual abuse. These programs were few in number and were quite different from one another: one, for example, was located in a probation department, another in a child welfare department, and a third in a hospital-based rape crisis center. Although their theoretical orientations and practical designs had little in common, they were all in agreement that it was essential to bring survivors together into groups. Inspired by these programs, these two authors set out to start a group for women survivors of incest. A colleague and mentor, Robert Ziegler, suggested adapting a recently developed model of time-limited psychotherapy (Mann, 1973) to a group design. And thus the TRG was created.

Throughout the 1980s, the group model was refined in consultation with a group of professional colleagues and peer group leaders from Incest Resources, a self-help organization. In addition, Janet Yassen, a colleague and one of the founders of the Boston Area Rape Crisis Center, provided supervision. The largest source of information about the group came from the clients themselves, who were interviewed 6 months postgroup to assess their own progress as well as provide data about what had and had not been helpful during the course of the group therapy (see Herman & Schatzow, 1984).

Within a short period of time, there was great demand for these groups. Judith Herman and Emily Schatzow were called upon to consult for other agencies that were trying to offer similar services and ran private trainings to teach the group model to other clinicians, using direct or videotaped observation wherever possible. They also began to offer the group model in the Department of Psychiatry at Cambridge Hospital, a community hospital in Cambridge, Massachusetts, where many clients reported histories of exposure to violence (Herman, 1986). Beginning in the mid-1980s, the Victims of Violence (VOV) Program at Cambridge Hospital became the primary locus of TRG offerings, and the original group model was adapted to reach a broader population of trauma survivors. Emily Schatzow, who served as coordinator of group services at the VOV Program for more than a decade, oversaw the adaptation of the model and supervised most of the groups. With VOV clinicians Phillip Brown and Melissa Coco, the model was also expanded to apply to a mixed male and female ("co-ed") membership.

In the years that followed, the TRG and the co-ed group were facilitated by many clinicians at the VOV Program, and co-leading these groups became an important component of the learning experience of the many psychiatry residents, psychology fellows, and social work fellows who came to the VOV Program for training. The impetus to document the TRG came from repeated positive feedback from both clients and clinicians about the helpful and rewarding experience of group participation and a growing view within the program that group therapy should be a treatment of choice for survivors of interpersonal trauma.

Translating a clinical model from an oral tradition to a written guide can be a daunting task. The process that led to the completion of this treatment guide was overseen by Michaela Mendelsohn, who directed the VOV research team from 2004 to 2009. Jocelyn Levitan, Melissa Coco, and Diya Kallivayalil provided administrative, clinical, and research input and support, respectively, for this project, although these roles frequently overlapped. The project would not have been completed without the collective contributions of all of the authors of this treatment guide.

Development of the guide proceeded in a number of stages. At the start, focus groups were conducted with the senior clinicians who had developed and adapted this group model to elucidate its key features. Then one 16-week group, co-led by clinicians with expertise in the model (Melissa Coco and Michaela Mendelsohn, supervised by Judith Herman), was videotaped, transcribed, and studied to provide many of the clinical examples included in the following chapters. Based on the information gathered from focus groups and the demonstration group, a first draft of the treatment guide was written.

Next, the draft was tested to determine whether it could serve as a reliable guide. Two group leaders new to implementation of the model (Diya Kallivayalil and Avivah Goldman, supervised by Barbara Hamm) used a draft of the treatment guide to conduct a second videotaped 16-week pilot group. Clients participating in both groups completed a battery of self-report measures and a semistructured interview to assess psychological symptoms and recovery status before and after the group. Group members and leaders were also asked for feedback about their experiences at the treatment's completion. The outcome data were collected, managed, and analyzed by Michaela Mendelsohn, Diya Kallivayalil, and Jocelyn

Levitan. On the basis of these data as well as observation of the pilot group, the treatment guide was revised to improve its clarity and usefulness.

Additional focus groups were conducted with clinicians experienced in the use of the model to gather information about supervision, and supervisory sessions from both groups were also transcribed. The focus groups and supervision transcripts formed the basis of the chapter on supervision. Finally, a draft of the revised treatment guide was circulated among the clinicians who had co-led the groups or participated in the focus groups, and their feedback was incorporated. The draft guide was expanded for publication with a more extensive literature review, further explanation of key components of the group model, material on adapting it to other treatment populations, integration of more clinical examples, and inclusion of treatment outcome data.

Chapter 1 of this book provides an overview of the prevalence and impact of interpersonal violence. It also reviews current psychosocial treatments, including individual and group therapy models, and locating the TRG approach in this framework. Chapter 2 reviews the format and structure of the group as a whole and of each session. Chapter 3 provides a detailed description of considerations in preparing to conduct a group and in screening potential group members to ensure a good match between the group and the client's treatment needs. Chapters 4–6 describe in depth the implementation of the group model in the introductory, goal work, and concluding phases, respectively. Since it is essential that group leaders utilize some form of supervision or consultation when conducting the TRG, Chapter 7 provides a guide for the supervisor. Chapter 8 outlines considerations in adapting this group model to other settings and populations and describes two examples of successfully implemented adaptations. Finally, Chapter 9 presents preliminary treatment outcome data from quantitative and qualitative research studies of TRG implementation. The appendices contain forms and other material that are useful in member recruitment, group preparations and screening, and implementation of the group.

The primary purpose of this book is describing the key elements of conducting a group of this kind. However, the clinician is permitted considerable flexibility in the ways in which most of these elements can be implemented, based on personal style, clinical setting, and characteristics of the client population. Our collective experience with implementing this group treatment approach has been primarily with women survivors of interpersonal trauma. As a result, this guide is based on a women's group, and female pronouns are used to refer to group members and leaders. However, as is discussed in Chapter 8, this model has also been successfully applied in mixed-gender groups and is certainly suitable for implementation in a men's group, although leaders should be mindful of gender differences in traumatic experiences and subsequent responses.

The clinical material includes case descriptions and transcripts from actual clients as well as fictional examples. Where actual client material has been used, we have changed demographic information and other identifying details to preserve anonymity. Written consent was obtained from all clients who are directly quoted in the treatment guide. Clients who participated in screening sessions or research interviews and the groups used to develop this treatment guide consented to having their sessions video- and/or audiotaped.

This project and the group outcome research were approved by the Cambridge Health Alliance Institutional Review Board.

This book is the result of a collaborative effort that began over 30 years ago and involved input from many people. We are extremely grateful to the VOV staff and trainees who have conducted the TRG over the years and shared their thoughts and experiences with us. In particular, we would like to thank the following clinicians who have made instrumental contributions to this project, to the development of the TRG model, and/or to our thinking about group therapy for trauma survivors: Phillip Brown, Lois Glass, Avivah Goldman, Barbara Hamm, Mary Harvey, Maggie Jarmolowski, Shirley Moore, Sarah Muzzy, Sally O'Leary, Jayme Shorin, Janet Yassen, and Robin Zachary. We would also like to acknowledge Anna Cerio, Esther Reidler, and Caroline Silva for transcribing interviews and providing research assistance and Bernadette Louis for overall administrative support.

We are profoundly grateful to Wallis Annenberg and the Annenberg Foundation for generously funding the project that resulted in this treatment guide. Without timely support from Ms. Annenberg, we could never have undertaken this task. We are also grateful to the Sarah Haley Memorial Fund for an award to Melissa Coco that enabled her to work on this project.

Most of all, we are indebted to our group members from 1984 to the present time, whose struggles and successes inspired this work. We deeply appreciate the courage of the women who agreed to be videotaped and interviewed for the purpose of documenting this group in the interests of helping other survivors.

It is our hope that this book will facilitate the creation of many new groups, that clinicians will find it interesting, perhaps even inspiring, and that survivors who participate in these groups will experience the empowerment and liberation that come from a restored sense of community.

MICHAELA MENDELSOHN
JUDITH LEWIS HERMAN
EMILY SCHATZOW
MELISSA COCO
DIYA KALLIVAYALIL
JOCELYN LEVITAN

Contents

CHAPTER 1

Interpersonal Violence and Trauma Recovery

Group therapy provides the survivor of interpersonal violence with unparalleled opportunities to combat social isolation, connect with sources of resilience and self-esteem, and rebuild relational capacities. This treatment guide describes a time-limited approach to group treatment first developed over 25 years ago for women survivors of childhood sexual abuse. It has since been adapted by clinicians at the Victims of Violence Program of the Cambridge Health Alliance for a broader population of trauma survivors, both men and women. The Trauma Recovery Group (TRG) is one of the mainstays of our treatment program. It is our hope that this guide enables mental health clinicians working with similar clients in other settings to replicate this treatment approach.

Women and girls are most likely to be victims of crimes of interpersonal violence such as rape, sexual abuse, and battering; the perpetrators are most likely to be men. The majority of women who experience violence are abused by the people closest to them—intimate partners, family members, and other trusted people in their daily environment. In the lives of many women, violence is a pervasive, tenacious, and frequently occurring event. This is a worldwide phenomenon that crosses the lines of race, ethnicity, nationality and national origin, class, religion, age, and sexual orientation (Marin & Russo, 1999; United Nations Population Fund [UNFPA], 2000).

The model of treatment we describe in this book is based on a feminist understanding of gender-based violence. We view rape, sexual abuse, and battering not as random acts perpetrated by disturbed individuals but rather as expressions of male power that perpetuate the subordination of women. These abuses are deeply embedded in the psychology and the social structures of patriarchy, sanctioned by custom and tradition, and often enacted in a ritualized manner (as in the case of gang rape). We believe it is for this reason that these acts of violence are so rarely treated as crimes and so often are hidden, excused, or even condoned. It is also for this reason that the victims of these crimes are so frequently silenced, blamed, and shamed.

Because feminism is so often misunderstood, it is important to clarify what this word means to us. *Feminism*, as we understand it, is simply an extension of democratic and egalitarian principles to the condition of women. Feminist thinking is based on a tradition that affirms human rights to life, liberty, and dignity. It challenges authoritarian and hierarchical social structures of any kind, whether based on race, religion, class, caste, culture, or gender. It does not imply hostility toward men; on the contrary, a feminist vision affirms the benefits of equality for both women *and* men.

Since a feminist understanding of violence focuses on issues of power, it is also directly relevant to the experiences of many male survivors of interpersonal violence, particularly survivors of sexual abuse or assault. In these instances also, most perpetrators are male. Boys and men who are victimized in this manner often interpret the experience as an assault on their gender identity, for in the rigid social codes of patriarchy to be sexually violated *is* to be "feminized." The gender confusion and humiliation that male survivors experience must be directly addressed in the process of recovery.

APPLYING FEMINIST PRINCIPLES TO TRAUMA RECOVERY

The idea of social equality between men and women may seem simple in principle, but realizing it in practice is a profoundly complex task. The subordinate condition of women is deeply ensconced in social customs, both in the public sphere of work and political participation and in the private sphere of sex, reproduction, and child care (Mitchell, 1966, 1971). Inevitably, therefore, patterns of dominance and subordination have also become deeply ingrained in the psychology of men and women (Miller, 1976). The idea that women's rights are human rights has only relatively recently been recognized as an international principle (Convention on the Elimination of All Forms of Discrimination against Women [CEDAW], 1979). Even more recent is the recognition that violence against women and girls constitutes a form of sex discrimination and represents a serious obstacle to their enjoyment of fundamental freedoms and human rights, as elaborated in the Declaration on the Elimination of Violence Against Women, promulgated by the United Nations in 1992 (United Nations General Assembly, 1993).

Some years ago, the United Nations Human Rights Council designated an investigator to consider the causes and consequences of violence against women. After visiting many countries to study and review this global problem, the investigator recently submitted her report. She concluded that ending gender-based violence will not be a simple matter of law and law enforcement, but rather will require the empowerment of women in many spheres of life. In the broad feminist vision of this report, empowerment means not only access to education and economic resources such as housing, property, and the fruits of gainful labor (although these are essential) but also the ability to move beyond protectionist and honor-based patriarchal customs regarding gender roles and sex, toward a more affirmative acceptance of sexuality (Erturk, 2009). Thus, the feminist idea of empowerment, though very simple in principle, in practice seeks to accomplish nothing less than the radical transformation of social relations worldwide. This same feminist vision of empowerment guides our general approach to treating survivors of interpersonal violence, and its application to the TRG is discussed in further detail in Chapter 2.

The principles of feminism are the principles of democracy and human rights. Although these may seem like idealistic and abstract concepts, we believe that they have very concrete meanings in the daily life of women and men, boys and girls. We maintain that it is in the nature of human beings to resist domination and arbitrary rule. Human beings thrive when they are treated with dignity and respect and when they are given the opportunity to participate actively in the social, economic and political life of their communities. They suffer psychological harm when they are forced to submit to the will of others and subjected to violence or contempt.

In the following pages, we review the literature on the psychological effects of interpersonal violence and the therapeutic remedies that have been developed thus far. Virtually absent from these studies is any analysis of the social ecology of violence. Thus, for example, investigators may simply report that the prevalence of posttraumatic stress disorder (PTSD) for women in the United States is twice as high as for men (10.4% vs. 5.0%) without exploring the social causes of this remarkable fact (Kessler, Sonnega, Bromet, Hughes, & Nelson, 1995). Social and political conceptual thinking is generally lacking in the psychology literature that is the subject of our brief review; however, we return to our basic feminist analytical frame at the end of the chapter when we introduce the unique features of our TRG therapy model.

THE IMPACT OF INTERPERSONAL VIOLENCE: THE SCOPE OF THE PROBLEM

Interpersonal violence has profound and far-reaching consequences for individuals and society. While the mental health field has made great advances in understanding and treating posttraumatic reactions, the challenge remains to find ways of addressing the more pervasive and enduring effects of exposure to chronic interpersonal violence.

For the purposes of this book, we define *interpersonal violence* broadly as physical and/or sexual assault or abuse intentionally perpetrated by one or more persons on another. It may be experienced at any point in the lifespan as a single incident or be repeated. The perpetrator may be a family member, a friend, an acquaintance, or a stranger. These and other specifics influence the way interpersonal violence is experienced; however, a common unifying feature is that the violence is enacted in the context of a relationship. Typical examples include childhood physical and/or sexual abuse, intimate partner violence, and adult sexual assault.

Although other types of violent events such as motor vehicle accidents and natural disasters have some interpersonal components, the connection between the parties is typically more remote, and the event is usually the result of negligence rather than intention (as in the case of accidents) or is not of human design at all (as with natural disasters). There is considerable evidence that psychological trauma is most severe in response to events result-ing from human agency and intention (Charuvastra & Cloitre, 2008). While combat, war, and political violence are also interpersonal in character, these are typically public events that are experienced collectively.

Our focus in this book is on interpersonal violence in the private sphere. However, we are well aware of the profound impact of war and political violence, both on combatants and on civilians who have the misfortune to live in war zones (Krippner & McIntyre, 2003; Weathers, Litz, & Keane, 1995). In particular, as civilians are increasingly targeted during armed conflicts, gender-based violence has become a common problem of wartime as well as one of private life. Wholesale rape of civilian women by conquering armies or marauding "irregular" forces has been widely reported and has been specifically recognized by the United Nations as a war crime (Farley, 2008). Moreover, as women become integrated into fighting forces, they face increasing risk of sexual assault not only by enemy forces but also, sadly, by peers and officers in their own units. This phenomenon has become so widespread that a new term, *military sexual trauma* (MST), has been coined to describe it (Kimerling, Gima, Smith, Street, & Frayne, 2007). Although our experience with the TRG has been limited to civilian survivors, we believe this group could be readily adapted for survivors of interpersonal violence in war and civil conflict.

Prevalence of Interpersonal Violence

Interpersonal violence is alarmingly widespread in our society. The National Violence Against Women Survey (NVAWS; Tjaden & Thoennes, 2000), based on a random sample of 16,000 men and women, found that 17.6% of women and 3.0% of men reported having experienced an attempted or completed rape in their lifetime. More than half of the female victims and almost three-quarters of the male victims reported that they were younger than 18 years when they experienced their first attempted or completed rape. Lifetime physical assault was reported by 51.9% of women and 66.4% of men; for men, the most com-mon assailant was a stranger, while for women the most common assailant was an intimate partner or family member. Intimate partner violence was reported by 22.1% of women and 7.4% of men.

Another large survey, the Adverse Childhood Experiences Study (Edwards, Holden, Felitti, & Anda, 2003), found that 21.6% of a large sample of adults in a primary care setting reported having experienced childhood sexual abuse (25.1% of women and 17.5% of men), 20.6% reported having experienced childhood physical abuse (19.7% of women and 21.7% of men), and 14.0% reported witnessing domestic violence during childhood (15.3% of women and 12.3% of men).

Most recently, a very large survey of over 4 million men and approximately 186,000 women veterans who were outpatients within the VHA health care system found that 22% of the women and 1% of the men screened positive for military sexual trauma, defined as either sexual harassment or sexual assault. Both women and men who screened positive for MST were significantly more likely to have a service-connected disability. MST was also highly correlated with a number of serious mental health conditions, including PTSD, dissociative disorders, eating disorders, personality disorders, and substance abuse (Kimerling et al., 2007).

Survivors of interpersonal violence are disproportionately represented among people seeking mental health or substance abuse treatment. In a large study of clients with severe mental illness, Mueser et al. (2004) found that 84% (86% of men and 82% of women) reported exposure to physical assault and 52% (40% of men and 68% of women) reported exposure to sexual assault in their lifetime. Childhood sexual abuse has been reported among as many as 53% of female psychiatric inpatients and 30–50% of outpatients (Bryer, Nelson, Miller, & Krol, 1987; Jacobson, 1989; Jacobson & Richardson, 1987). Hien and Scheier (1996) found that 63% of women receiving inpatient alcohol and drug detoxification reported a history of childhood trauma (including direct physical or sexual abuse or witnessing extreme parental violence), 69.3% reported a history of adulthood intimate partner violence, and 57.4% reported a history of adulthood sexual assault or participation in sex-for-drug exchanges. In a study of women dually diagnosed with a substance use and mental health disorder, 84.9% reported physical abuse by a known person, 71.4% reported that they had been stalked or threatened, 72.6% reported having been raped, and 67.1% reported other unwanted sexual contact over the course of their lifetime (McHugo et al., 2005). Other groups that have been similarly identified as having rates of interpersonal victimization substantially higher than the general population include female veterans (Skinner et al., 2000; Zinzow, Grubaugh, Monnier, Suffoletta-Maierle, & Frueh, 2007), incarcerated men and women (Browne, Miller, & Maguin, 1999; Weeks & Widom, 1998), persons infected with HIV (Whetten et al., 2006), and homeless women (Browne & Bassuk, 1997; Zugazaga, 2004).

Impact of Interpersonal Violence

PTSD is the most commonly recognized disorder associated with exposure to trauma and violence (American Psychiatric Association, 1994). It may follow exposure to an event that involves serious threat of injury or death and subjective feelings of fear, helplessness, or horror. The symptoms of PTSD are organized into three clusters: (1) reexperiencing the trauma in such ways as intrusive thoughts, dreams, or flashbacks; (2) avoidance of stimuli associated with the trauma as well as general emotional numbing; and (3) increased arousal evidenced by such symptoms as hypervigilance, increased startle response, and irritability. The diagnostic category was initially informed by the experiences of war veterans, rape survivors, and concentration camp survivors. Subsequently, the occurrence of PTSD has been confirmed following exposure to a wide range of extreme life events (Keane, Marshall, & Taft, 2006). It also appears to be an acceptable classification for psychological reactions to severe stressors across a variety of cultural settings (Osterman & de Jong, 2007).

Recognition of PTSD represented a major step forward in the diagnosis and treatment of victims of trauma. However, the disorder as presently defined does not adequately capture the range and complexity of problems frequently reported by survivors of prolonged and/or repeated interpersonal violence (Briere & Jordan, 2004; Ford & Courtois, 2009; Herman, 1992a; van der Kolk, 1996). These survivors, both women and men, often manifest the symptoms of many other diagnoses besides PTSD, including mood disorders (Koss, Bailey, & Yuan,

2003; Neria et al., 2008), other anxiety disorders (David, Giron, & Mellman, 1995; Zlotnick et al., 2008), eating disorders (de Groot & Rodin, 1999; Wonderlich et al., 2001), substance abuse (Dube et al., 2003; Najavits, Weiss, & Shaw, 1997), dissociation (Chu & Dill, 1990; Putnam, Guroff, Silberman, Barban, & Post, 1986), somatization and conversion disorders (Roelofs, Keijsers, Hoogduin, Näring, & Moene, 2002; Stein et al., 2004), sexual dysfunction (Courtois, 1997; Sarwer & Durlak, 1996), and personality disorders (Herman, Perry, & van der Kolk, 1989; Ogata, Silk, & Goodrich, 1990; Westen, Ludolf, & Misle, 1990).

Prolonged and repeated interpersonal violence, particularly childhood abuse, has been associated with increased risk of self-injurious and suicidal behaviors (Boudewyn & Liem, 1995; Briere & Runtz, 1993; Dube et al., 2001; van der Kolk, Perry, & Herman, 1991). Similarly, increased risk of suicide attempts has been found among victims of domestic violence (McCauley et al., 1995; Thompson et al., 1999). Childhood physical or sexual abuse is a strong predictor of revictimization in adulthood (Classen, Palesh, & Aggarwal, 2005; Coid et al., 2001; Rich, Combs-Lane, Resnick, & Kilpatrick, 2004). Survivors of chronic interpersonal violence are also more vulnerable to a variety of physical health problems (Leserman, 2005; Romans, Belaise, Martin, Morris, & Raffi, 2002; Walker et al., 1999).

These findings, coupled with accumulated clinical observations, have led to an expanded conceptualization of the long-term effects of prolonged and repeated interpersonal violence. Herman (1992a) formulated the concept of complex PTSD to describe three broad areas of disturbance commonly reported in the literature and observed in clinical practice but not adequately captured by a simple diagnosis of PTSD. First, survivors present a complicated and tenacious symptom picture with multiple complaints, most commonly including somatization, dissociation, and affective dysregulation (van der Kolk et al., 1996). Second, they display characteristic personality changes, including relational difficulties and disturbances of identity. Third, they are vulnerable to repeated harm, either self-inflicted or perpetrated by others.

van der Kolk, Roth, Pelcovitz, Sunday, and Spinazzola (2005) have proposed the classification of disorders of extreme stress not otherwise specified (DESNOS) to summarize the multiple domains of symptomatology associated with chronic interpersonal trauma. These include alterations in

1. regulation of affect and impulses (e.g., suicidal and self-destructive behavior, risk taking),
2. attention and consciousness (i.e., dissociation),
3. biological self-regulation (i.e., somatization, e.g., chronic pain, conversion symptoms),
4. self-perceptions (e.g., feeling damaged, shame),
5. perceptions of the perpetrator (e.g., idealization, adopting distorted beliefs),
6. relationships with others (e.g., trust difficulties, revictimization), and
7. systems of meaning (e.g., feelings of despair, loss of sustaining beliefs).

Field trials conducted during the development of the fourth edition of the *Diagnostic and Statistical Manual of Mental Disorders* (DSM-IV) confirmed that the development of DES-

NOS was associated with experiencing early interpersonal trauma, younger age of trauma onset, and longer exposure to traumatic events. These symptoms were found to occur in addition to PTSD and were more strongly associated with treatment seeking than straightforward PTSD (van der Kolk et al., 2005). Studies with civilian and military samples have confirmed that DESNOS is most likely to occur following trauma in early childhood (when many self-capacities are formed) and following interpersonal violence (Ford & Courtois, 2009). In DSM-IV (American Psychiatric Association, 1994), the symptoms of complex PTSD are listed as associated features of PTSD. Debate is currently under way regarding the best way to conceptualize the enduring effects of chronic interpersonal trauma in DSM-5, due to be released in 2013.

Regardless of how the psychological effects are categorized, it is clear that they are pervasive and far-reaching. In addition to the enormous pain and suffering experienced by individual survivors and those close to them, there are significant social and economic costs associated with the high rates of such exposure to interpersonal violence. A number of studies show that traumatized men and women have high rates of medical and psychiatric service utilization (Gillock, Zayfert, Hegel, & Ferguson, 2005; Stein, McQuaid, Pedrelli, Lenox, McCahill, 2000; Switzer et al., 1999), thus contributing to strains on the health care delivery system. Trauma exposure and PTSD have also been associated with difficulties in maintaining employment and functioning effectively in work settings (Izutsu, Shibuya, Tsutsumi, Konishi, & Kawamura, 2008; Kimerling et al., 2009), thereby making an economic impact. Furthermore, there is an abundance of evidence on the impact of trauma on parenting and the transmission of trauma from one generation to the next (Cohen, Hien, & Batchelder, 2008; Lauterbach et al., 2007; Noll, Trickett, Harris, & Putnam, 2009). There is thus a pressing need for appropriate treatments to address the enduring effects of interpersonal violence.

PSYCHOSOCIAL TREATMENTS FOR THE EFFECTS OF INTERPERSONAL VIOLENCE

Individual Psychotherapy

To date, most empirical studies of treatment outcomes for survivors of interpersonal violence focus on symptoms of simple PTSD without any of the complicating factors that are so commonly observed in survivors of prolonged and repeated violence. Within these limited parameters, the psychosocial treatments for PTSD with the strongest empirical support are cognitive-behavioral therapy and eye movement desensitization and reprocessing (Bradley, Greene, Russ, Dutra, & Westen, 2005; Resick, Monson, & Gutner, 2007). In a meta-analysis of 26 studies conducted between 1980 and 2003, Bradley et al. (2005) found that 67% of clients who complete one of these brief psychotherapy protocols and 56% of those who enter treatment (whether or not they complete it) no longer meet the criteria for PTSD. They caution, however, that stringent exclusion criteria and failure to address polysymptomatic presentations limit the generalizability of these efficacy studies to clients seen in clinical practice. While other approaches, such psychodynamic psychotherapy, are frequently utilized by practitioners in treating trauma survivors, they lend themselves less readily to empirical study, and outcome data is therefore limited.

Cognitive-Behavioral Therapy

There are a number of effective cognitive-behavioral therapies (CBTs) for PTSD that vary in the extent to which they rely on such behavioral techniques as exposure or relaxation training and cognitive restructuring. Three commonly utilized approaches are exposure therapy, anxiety management training, and cognitive therapy. In addition, one very promising cognitive-behavioral treatment protocol has been developed specifically for survivors of complex trauma.

EXPOSURE THERAPY

Applied to PTSD treatment, exposure therapy typically involves repeated confrontation with memories of the trauma (imaginal exposure) and with trauma-related situations that give rise to unrealistic fears (*in vivo* exposure; Zoellner, Fitzgibbons, & Foa, 2001). Exposure may be graded (e.g., using systematic desensitization) or may involve implosion or flooding (Solomon & Johnson, 2002). Repeated exposures lead to habituation and a decrease in anxiety associated with trauma-related stimuli. Some approaches include the provision of new information that is incompatible with the existing fear structure of PTSD, promoting change in irrational beliefs about threat. Prolonged exposure (PE; Foa & Rothbaum, 1998) is an example of such a treatment approach. PE involves two initial sessions of information gathering and treatment planning, followed by seven sessions in which the client imagines the trauma as vividly as possible and repeatedly describes it aloud in the present tense. An audiotape is made of the client's narrative, and homework involves listening daily to the trauma narrative as well as planned exposure to feared but objectively safe situations to promote accommodation of corrective information.

There is extensive evidence attesting to the effectiveness of PE and other exposure-based techniques in reducing symptoms of PTSD (Keane et al., 2006; Nemeroff et al., 2006; Rothbaum, Meadows, Resick, & Foy, 2000); however, these treatments are applied relatively rarely by clinicians in real-world settings (Cook, Schnurr, & Foa, 2004). Concerns have been raised about high treatment dropout rates (e.g., Schottenbauer, Glass, Arnkoff, Tendick, & Gray, 2008). Moreover, practitioners may be quite appropriately reluctant to implement exposure therapies (which at least temporarily increase anxiety) with complexly traumatized clients suffering from poor impulse and affect regulation skills as well as high-risk behaviors such as substance abuse or self-injury.

ANXIETY MANAGEMENT TECHNIQUES

Anxiety management techniques (AMTs) refer to a variety of procedures for reducing trauma-related anxiety and associated affect, based on the idea that pathological anxiety is a result of deficits in coping skills. Examples include biofeedback, relaxation training, breathing retraining, guided self-dialogue, distraction, social skills training, and anger management training (Keane et al., 2006; Solomon & Johnson, 2002). Stress inoculation training (SIT) is the anxiety management program most frequently studied in the treatment of PTSD. Based on Meichenbaum's work, it was adapted by Kilpatrick, Veronen, and Resnick (1982) for adult rape survivors. It incorporates a number of components that include education, relaxation, breathing control, role playing, cognitive restructuring, covert modeling, and thought stopping. A number of empirical studies have demonstrated the effectiveness of SIT and other AMTs in reducing PTSD symptoms, although the effects appear less marked and sustained than for exposure-based treatments (Foa, 1997; Nemeroff et al., 2006; Zoellner et al., 2001).

COGNITIVE APPROACHES

Cognitive models of PTSD theorize that the central problem lies in the survivor's inability to process the trauma, resulting in distress when confronted with internal and external cues and avoidance of traumatic reminders. Cognitive therapy helps the client cope with the traumatic memories and associated negative thoughts and expectations (Tucker & Trautman, 2000). Originally developed for women with rape-related PTSD, cognitive processing therapy (CPT; Resick & Schnicke, 1993) combines aspects of exposure therapy, AMT, and cognitive therapy. After the client's initial orientation to treatment, exposure sessions involve writing and reading trauma narratives. The cognitive therapy component involves addressing key cognitive distortions associated with the traumatic event. CPT targets five schemas frequently disrupted by trauma, namely, safety, trust, power and control, self-esteem, and intimacy. Although the research literature is smaller than for behaviorally oriented treatments, a number of studies have supported the effectiveness of cognitive therapies for PTSD (Resick, 2001). One large trial of CPT found results comparable with prolonged exposure, with better scores on certain guilt-related measures (Resick, Nishith, Weaver, Astin, & Feuer, 2002). Efforts have been made to adapt CPT to other traumatized groups, including survivors of childhood sexual abuse, with initial studies indicating good effects (Chard 2005; House, 2006).

SKILLS TRAINING IN AFFECT AND INTERPERSONAL REGULATION WITH MODIFIED PROLONGED EXPOSURE

Skills training in affect and interpersonal regulation with modified prolonged exposure (STAIR-MPE; Cloitre, Cohen, & Koenen, 2006) is a very promising example of individual cognitive-behavioral therapy specifically modified to meet the needs of survivors of chronic interpersonal trauma. STAIR-MPE was developed based on the recognition that affective dysregulation and interpersonal deficits frequently cause survivors of complex trauma as much distress as their PTSD symptoms but are frequently unaddressed by standard treatments. STAIR-MPE is a manualized phase-oriented CBT that draws on skills training from dialectical behavior therapy and the success of exposure therapy in ameliorating symptoms of PTSD. The first phase of treatment consists of eight sessions designed to teach the client skills for mood regulation, distress tolerance, and emotional management in interpersonal contexts. The second phase involves eight sessions of traumatic memory exposure therapy modified to prevent cognitive or affective dysregulation, also referred to as narrative story telling. Cloitre, Koenen, Cohen, and Han (2002) found that women who received STAIR-MPE showed a significant improvement in dealing with affect regulation problems, interpersonal skills deficits, and PTSD symptoms relative to a wait-list control group; these gains were maintained and some were enhanced at 3- and 6-month follow-up. Development of a positive therapeutic alliance and improvement in negative mood regulation during the first phase were significant predictors of PTSD reductions during the second (exposure) phase.

Eye Movement Desensitization and Reprocessing

Eye movement desensitization and reprocessing (EMDR; Shapiro, 1989) combines saccadic eye movements with imaginal exposure and cognitive processing. The client is instructed to move his or her eyes back and forth, tracking the therapist's finger for about 15–20 seconds while maintaining an image of the traumatic event. The client reports the negative self-cognitions, emotions, and physical sensations that emerge. This process is repeated until the client reports a decrease in anxiety. The reprocessing phase involves the installation of more positive thoughts (Solomon & Johnson, 2002). EMDR has been associated with some controversy, as claims about the centrality of saccadic eye movements have been criticized as lacking a theoretical and scientific basis (Keane et al., 2006). There is a considerable body of literature supporting the effectiveness of EMDR in reducing PTSD symptoms, although it does not appear to be more effective than other exposure-based treatments, and the eye movements do not appear to be integral to the treatment (Davidson & Parker, 2001; Zoellner et al., 2001). There have been a number of anecdotal descriptions of the application of EMDR to complexly traumatized clients (e.g., Korn & Leeds, 2002; Twombly, 2000).

Psychodynamic Psychotherapy

Several models of brief psychodynamic psychotherapy have been proposed for the treatment of PTSD, although there have been very few controlled outcome studies regarding their effectiveness. Horowitz (1997) described a 12-session treatment model consisting of three phases: (1) developing a working alliance, during which the client also tells his or her trauma story; (2) "working through," which involves exploration and clarification of the underlying beliefs, emotions, themes, and defenses that make the trauma difficult to integrate; and (3) dealing with the loss associated with the trauma and the ending of therapy. Psychodynamic components of the model include bringing conflicts into conscious awareness, using the therapeutic relationship, and analyzing defenses. The treatment additionally provides education about the effects of trauma and coping while also focusing on trauma-related intrapersonal and interpersonal themes. Brom, Kleber, and Defares (1989) conducted a randomized controlled trial comparing an earlier version of this treatment approach to systematic desensitization and hypnotherapy. Some 60% of all treated clients versus 26% of untreated clients showed clinically significant improvements. It was found that psychodynamic therapy resulted in greater reduction of avoidance symptoms, while the other two treatments led to greater decreases in intrusive symptoms. Participants in psychodynamic therapy showed less improvement immediately posttreatment but had improved to the same level as participants in other groups at 3-month follow-up. This model was developed for survivors of a single traumatic event, and it has been noted that it is not well suited to clients with chronic or complex PTSD, who may require longer-term or more comprehensive treatment (Krupnick, 2002). However, it has been suggested that psychodynamic approaches in general may be particularly well suited to the diffuse sequelae of complex trauma that are not well targeted by empirically supported treatments that focus on reducing PTSD symptoms alone (Schottenbauer, Glass, Arnkoff, & Gray, 2008).

Other individual therapy approaches to the treatment of PTSD that have not been subject to extensive empirical validation include supportive therapy, hypnotherapy, interpersonal therapy, and eclectic therapy. Over recent years, partly in response to the unaddressed treatment needs of complex trauma survivors, a number of new treatments have been developed or adapted specifically for this population. These include internal family systems therapy (Schwartz, 1995), accelerated experiential–dynamic psychotherapy (Fosha, 2000), and sensorimotor psychotherapy (Ogden, Minton, & Pain, 2006). The reader is referred to Courtois and Ford (2009) for a detailed description of these and other emerging approaches.

As reviewed above, there are many clinical descriptions and outcome studies as well as a number of published treatment guidelines for the treatment patients with simple PTSD (e.g., Benedek, Friedman, Zatzick, & Ursano, 2009; Foa, Keane, & Friedman, 2000). Unfortunately, these studies typically do not address the DESNOS/complex PTSD symptoms described earlier. Indeed, many specifically *exclude* individuals with severe comorbid psychopathology, that is those with more complex presentations (Bradley et al., 2005; Spinazzola, Blaustein, & van der Kolk, 2005). Thus, although there is a growing literature describing clinical interventions with complexly traumatized clients, there are relatively few empirical studies and no official guidelines for this population. Courtois, Ford, and Cloitre (2009) note that while existing recommendations for the treatment of PTSD may often be applicable to patients with complex traumatic stress disorders, they cannot be expected to fully ameliorate the range of self-regulation problems that originate from developmentally adverse interpersonal trauma.

Because patients suffering from complex PTSD typically experience multiple co-occurring problems, good treatment is likely to be multimodal (Briere & Jordan, 2004; Courtois et al., 2009), involving some combination of psychopharmacology, individual, family and/or group psychotherapy, and nonclinical or community-based interventions (e.g., advocacy). It is important that care be coordinated and that there be good communication and collaboration among all the professionals involved in the patient's care to prevent duplication, fragmentation, and splitting. Moreover, we would propose that applications of known treatment methods be informed by an understanding of the concept of recovery stages.

A Stage-Based Model of Trauma Recovery

A phase-oriented approach to trauma treatment has been increasingly adopted with growing awareness of the complex presentation and needs of many trauma survivors (Ford, Courtois, Steele, van der Hart, & Nijenhuis, 2005). Herman (1992b) was the first to synthesize clinical observations and research literature into an understanding of recovery from trauma as unfolding over three progressive stages. This model of recovery is based on the idea that helplessness, meaninglessness, and disconnection from oneself and others are central components of the experience of interpersonal trauma. Empowerment and the creation of new meanings and connections are thus key aspects of the recovery process.

Stage 1 of recovery involves the establishment of *safety*. This focus may begin with the body (e.g., regulation of such basic functions as sleep and eating; management of intrusive PTSD symptoms; control over self-destructive behaviors). It then proceeds outward to the environment (e.g., establishment of a safe and stable living situation; attention to such issues as work and income). Only when safety is established can recovery move to the next stage, where the focus is on *remembrance, integration, and mourning*. The healing work of Stage 2 involves carefully paced in-depth exploration of the traumatic experiences, with the goal of integrating memory, affect, and cognition rather than simply facilitating catharsis. This stage inevitably involves a period of intense grief and mourning during which the survivor is sustained by his or her connections to the therapist and peers, the hope of building new and more adaptive relationships, and the creation of new meaning within the traumatic experiences. Stage 3 of recovery involves *reconnecting with others* through the process of establishing mutual nonexploitative relationships. The survivor may have to renegotiate the boundaries and limits of long-standing relationships, particularly those that have been abusive (Herman, 1992b; Lebowitz, Harvey, & Herman, 1993). Progression through the stages of recovery is not necessarily a linear process; individuals may move back and forth between phases (e.g., in response to a current crisis or traumatic reminder), and issues addressed in each phase are often recapitulated and elaborated in subsequent phases (Courtois et al., 2009; Ford et al., 2005).

An important implication of this view of trauma recovery is that treatment must be stage-appropriate in order to be helpful and effective. Early-stage interventions are thus focused on symptom mastery, stabilization, and the establishment of basic routines of self-care as well as on developing a treatment alliance, which can be predictably complicated with clients who have experienced relational trauma. The processing and integration of trauma memories is the hallmark of second-stage treatment; Courtois et al. (2009, p. 93) describe this task as the "safe self-reflective disclosure of traumatic memories and associated reactions in the form of progressively elaborated and coherent autobiographical narrative." The third stage of recovery typically involves efforts to expand the individual's social network, range of activities, and self-definition beyond that of trauma survivor, and may include nonclinical "interventions" such as increased community involvement and social activism.

Ford et al. (2005) identify five overarching treatment principles that are relevant throughout phase-oriented treatment of complex trauma:

1. Treatment should enhance the client's ability to manage extreme states of emotional arousal.
2. Treatment should enhance the client's sense of personal control and self-efficacy.
3. Treatment should assist the client in maintaining an adequate level of functioning consistent with his or her past and current lifestyle and circumstances.
4. Treatment should enhance the client's ability to approach and master, rather than avoid, internal states and external events that trigger posttraumatic stress symptoms.

5. Therapists must be aware of and effectively manage both their clients' transferential reactions and their own countertransference.

It is notable that this review of current individual treatment methods makes no reference to the social and political context in which violence occurs. We consider this a major deficiency. Without this broader perspective, survivors of interpersonal violence may remain isolated and trapped in the particulars of their experience without fully understanding the commonalities of their suffering. One of the best ways to foster the development of this broader perspective is to bring patients together into groups.

Group Therapy for Survivors of Interpersonal Trauma

A primary effect of interpersonal trauma is the disruption of social relatedness and attendant isolation of the victim. Survivors of gender-based violence, in particular, suffer from the secrecy, shame, and stigma that are the predictable social consequences of this form of violation. These acutely painful psychological states have been clinically observed among survivors of rape (Koss & Harvey, 1991), child sexual abuse (Herman & Schatzow, 1984), and domestic violence (Walker, 2000). They are also seen in combat veterans, particularly when community support for their fighting mission is lacking (Lifton, 1973).

Impairments in attachment and relational capacities have been repeatedly noted in studies of adult survivors of childhood abuse (Briere & Rickards, 2007; Cloitre, Miranda, Stovall-McClough, & Han, 2005; van der Kolk et al., 2005). In addition, many symptoms of PTSD such as avoidance, numbing, and irritability or anger outbursts are interpersonal in nature, making it difficult for survivors to connect with others (Pearlman & Courtois, 2005). There is abundant literature highlighting both the buffering effects of social support and the detrimental impact of its absence following exposure to trauma (Charuvastra & Cloitre, 2008); yet, the very nature of interpersonal trauma make this resource difficult to access.

By providing a safe and structured relational context for healing, group therapy provides a unique opportunity to restore social connections while also addressing the deleterious impact of interpersonal trauma on the survivor's experience of self in relationships. Groups provide survivors with an experience of both commonality and belonging and reduce feelings of isolation and alienation (Herman, 1992b). They provide opportunities for resiliencies among group members to be noticed and utilized, and also they promote a sense of pride by enabling members to share coping skills and help one another. They foster self-esteem as survivors learn to value themselves by establishing connections with valued others and experiencing their acceptance (Harney & Harvey, 1999). Group therapy provides an excellent environment for repairing the cognitive schemas for safety, trust/dependency, independence, power, self-esteem, and intimacy that are often disrupted by psychological trauma (Allen & Bloom, 1994). By providing a felt experience of reciprocal relationships marked by caring and compassion, group therapy can empower survivors to seek out safe and affirming relationships in their lives outside of group, functioning as an "ecological bridge to new community" (Mendelsohn, Zachary, & Harney, 2007, p. 227).

Over the past 25 years, mental health professionals have proposed and investigated a variety of group interventions for trauma survivors that vary in such dimensions as their duration, structure, and focus. Foy et al. (2001) identify three main orientations to group treatment with trauma survivors: supportive, cognitive-behavioral, and psychodynamic approaches. Supportive groups represent a "covering" approach, where emphasis is placed on addressing current life issues. In contrast, both cognitive-behavioral and psychodynamic groups represent an "uncovering" approach, as they are designed to address participants' traumatic experiences and memories directly. While they differ in regard to their underlying formulations of symptom etiology and maintenance, the three approaches share several common features: membership is relatively homogeneous, the traumatic experience is acknowledged and validated, traumatic responses are normalized, and a nonjudgmental stance is adopted toward behavior required for survival when the trauma occurred. Furthermore, the presence of others with a similar traumatic history dispels the notion that therapy cannot be helpful because the therapist has not shared the traumatic experience.

Outcome studies have focused on a variety of therapy groups for trauma survivors, many of which are methodologically limited (e.g., small sample size, absence of control or comparison groups, unstandardized assessment measures), and there is currently no strong evidence as to the superiority of one model over others (Fritch & Lynch, 2008). Based on a comprehensive review of empirical studies of group psychotherapy for adult trauma survivors, Foy et al. (2000) found that, regardless of the specific approach, group psychotherapy was associated with favorable outcomes in a wide range of symptom domains. Abatement of posttraumatic stress and depression were the most commonly noted outcomes, but efficacy was also demonstrated for other symptoms, including increased self-esteem and reduced dissociation, anxiety, fear, and global distress.

Beneficial effects have also been found in studies focusing specifically on victims of interpersonal trauma (primarily adult survivors of childhood sexual abuse) and including a wide variety of group treatment approaches such as problem solving (Richter, Snider, & Gorey, 1997), affect management (Zlotnick et al., 1997), psychoeducation (Lubin, Loris, Burt, & Johnson, 1998), body-oriented interventions (Westbury & Tutty, 1999), cognitive processing therapy (Chard, 2005), trauma-focused therapy (Classen, Koopman, Nevill-Manning, & Speigel, 2001), and process groups (Hazzard, Rogers, & Angert, 1993). Commonly reported improvements involve reductions in PTSD symptoms (e.g., Lubin et al., 1998), depression (e.g., Morgan & Cummings, 1999), and dissociation (e.g., Bradley & Follingstad, 2003) as well as increases in self-esteem and internal locus of control (e.g., Hazzard et al., 2003).

Applying a Stage-Based Approach to Group Treatment

Applied to group therapy, a stage-based model of trauma treatment implies that different types of groups will be appropriate for survivors at each stage of recovery. The characteristics of therapy groups for survivors in the three recovery stages are summarized in Table 1.1.

Stage 1 groups are designed for clients whose primary needs involve the establishment of safety, stability, and self-care. These groups emphasize the development of behavioral,

TABLE 1.1. Three Group Models

Group characteristic	Stage of recovery		
	Stage 1	Stage 2	Stage 3
Therapeutic task	Safety	Remembrance and mourning	Reconnection
Time orientation	Present	Past and present	Past, present, and future
Focus	Self-care	Trauma	Interpersonal relationships
Membership	Homogeneous	Homogeneous	Heterogeneous
Boundaries	Flexible and inclusive	Closed	Stable, slow turnover
Cohesion	Moderate	Very high	High
Conflict tolerance	Low	Low	High
Time limit	Open-ended or repeating	Fixed limit	Open-ended
Structure	Didactic	Goal-directed	Unstructured
Example	Twelve-step program	Survivor group	Interpersonal

Note. From Herman (1992b). Copyright 1992. Adapted by permission of Basic Books, a member of the Perseus Book Group.

cognitive, and psychosocial skills for managing symptoms and caring for oneself appropriately. They may have a didactic component. They are present-focused and may actively discourage significant disclosure of trauma histories to protect group members from becoming overwhelmed (Harney & Harvey, 1999). In Foy et al.'s (2001) classification, these would be considered either supportive or cognitive-behavioral groups.

Once safety and self-care are reasonably well established, symptoms are under a comfortable degree of control, social supports are reliable, and life circumstances are relatively stable, survivors ready to participate in a trauma-focused group in which the group members "bear witness" to one another's stories. The focus of these groups is the integration of the traumatic past with clients' present lives. In Foy et al.'s (2001) classification, many such groups employ cognitive-behavioral techniques such as prolonged exposure; others have evolved from variants of the psychodynamic tradition. Their feature in common is to directly confront the trauma narrative. We characterize these as Stage 2 groups.

Groups for survivors in Stage 3 of recovery generally address specific residual problems such as difficulties in sexual relationships, in which case a behavioral approach might be appropriate. Alternatively, they may focus on resolving remaining difficulties in interpersonal relationships; these problems are typically addressed in classic psychodynamic psychotherapy groups. In either case, we recommend that survivors in Stage 3 participate in a group with a relatively *heterogeneous* membership. Having integrated their past trauma and overcome the attendant shame and isolation, survivors will likely find a sense of community with a *wider* range of people (Herman, 1992b).

Manualized Group Treatments for Complex PTSD

Three existing manualized group treatment models have been developed for the same population that inspired the creation of the TRG, that is, female survivors of interpersonal trauma who present with symptoms of complex PTSD. These models are trauma recovery and empowerment (TREM; Harris, 1998), Seeking Safety (SS; Najavits, 2002), and trauma-centered group psychotherapy (TCGP) for women (Lubin & Johnson, 2008). First, we consider how each treatment approach fits within a "stage of recovery" model, and then we provide a brief overview of the TRG by discussing the ways in which it is similar to the other models and the ways in which it is unique.

TRAUMA RECOVERY AND EMPOWERMENT

TREM (Harris, 1998) was developed at a private not-for-profit mental health clinic in downtown Washington, DC. Designed to serve poor and socially marginalized women with histories of childhood physical and sexual abuse, the group combines basic education about the impact of trauma and feminist consciousness raising with skills building. The group format was developed both for practical (i.e., cost-effectiveness) and for therapeutic reasons; the group is envisioned as a "healing community" for women whose "core connections" to family, community, and self have been abruptly severed by trauma. Some 33 topics are covered in weekly meetings. Each topic is introduced with a brief clinical rationale, a set of goals, a series of questions to be posed to the group, and an experiential exercise. This is a clear-cut "Stage 1" group model, according to our stage-based formulation. The treatment may be adapted for male trauma survivors and for special populations including women with chronic mental illness and incarcerated women. There is one published outcome study of a modified version of TREM implemented in a residential substance abuse program. In this study, Toussaint, VanDeMark, Bornemann, and Graeber (2007) found that women who participated in TREM showed significantly better outcomes than those receiving treatment-as-usual on trauma-related symptoms, although not on alcohol or drug use.

SEEKING SAFETY

SS (Najavits, 2002) was designed as a treatment for clients with dual diagnoses of PTSD and substance abuse. Based primarily on a CBT model, it also draws on "some of the wisdom of psychodynamic therapy" and "strong respect for twelve-step and other self-help traditions" (p. viii). Twenty-five topics are addressed, and with each topic the client is asked to identify a safe coping skill relevant to both PTSD and substance abuse. The SS treatment can be conducted on either an individual or a group basis. This model explicitly recognizes the concept of recovery stages, and it is designed as a "Stage 1" intervention. Originally developed for women, it has been adapted for men as well. There are a number of studies supporting the effectiveness of SS in reducing trauma-related symptoms and substance use (Desai, Harpaz-Rotem, Najavits, & Rosenheck, 2008; Hien, Cohen, Miele, Litt, & Capstick, 2004; Najavits, Weiss, Shaw, & Muenz, 1998).

TRAUMA-CENTERED GROUP PSYCHOTHERAPY

TCGP (Lubin & Johnson, 2008) was designed specifically to address the interpersonal effects of trauma. The group has a firm psychoeducational structure, with 16 weekly sessions, each with a lecture topic, handouts, and homework assignments, followed by a "graduation ceremony" to which clients may invite friends or family members. The group discussion that follows each lecture is designed to evoke and then correct "traumatic schemas" as clients share their trauma memories. According to our recovery-stage formulations, this group is something of a "hybrid," combining the didactic structure of a Stage 1 group and the "exposure" features of a Stage 2 group. Originally developed for women, it has also been adapted for men and for special populations, including veterans and women with concurrent PTSD and substance abuse. An uncontrolled study of this treatment approach found significant posttreatment reductions in PTSD and depression that were sustained at 6-month follow-up (Lubin et al., 1998).

The Trauma Recovery Group

We come, finally, to the TRG. Our model of group treatment is designed to include survivors of all forms of interpersonal violence, including those who have been subjected to prolonged and repeated incidents of violence, either in childhood or throughout the adult lifespan. Unlike most other groups designed to address the needs of survivors of prolonged and repeated violence, this is a Stage 2 *trauma-focused* group. The central task of the group is the "uncovering" or "exposure" of the trauma story, with all of its secrets. However, this story telling is undertaken not for its own sake but rather to further an experience of active mastery in affiliation with other survivors. It is undertaken also as an implicit exercise in social and political consciousness-raising. As group members discover the commonalities in their experiences of interpersonal violence, they gain a broader understanding of the social context that permits such endemic violence to flourish. Feelings of "condemned isolation" (Miller, 1990) give way to feelings of mutual empathy and acceptance, while feelings of helpless rage and paralyzing terror give way to feelings of righteous indignation—first on behalf of others and only then on each survivor's own behalf.

With a sense of righteous outrage comes the wish to right social wrongs and a desire to move from enforced passivity to active empowerment. All group members are therefore asked to identify a personal goal related to the trauma that might be too difficult to contemplate in isolation but that might be possible to accomplish with the support of the group. This *goal orientation* provides a focus for each member's work in the group.

The TRG is always *time-limited* in order to contain the emotional intensity of trauma-focused work and provide an impetus for pursuing and achieving short-term goals related to the broader task of recovery. The duration has ranged from 10 weeks to as long as 32 weeks, most commonly running for 16 weeks. Groups begin with introductions and ground rules, progress through goal definition and the sharing of trauma stories, and then proceed to the achievement of goals. Groups end with a termination process involving review and feedback celebrating members' accomplishments. Group sessions are structured by the technique of *time sharing*, which ensures equal participation and mutuality. Another key feature of the TRG is *supportive process*, with emphasis on learning to give and receive empathic feedback. The group strives to create an environment in which members can experience safe attachment as well as use interpersonal interactions as opportunities for growth and mastery where relevant to their treatment goals. We strongly recommend *co-leadership* of the group for both practical reasons and the opportunities provided by this arrangement to model an adult caretaking relationship based on reciprocity, cooperation, and mutual respect. These characteristics and their implementation are described in greater detail in the following chapters.

Although originally developed in a private practice setting, the TRG has been adapted and used successfully in the outpatient psychiatry department of a large public hospital serving a highly diverse and largely impoverished population. Preliminary outcome studies (detailed in Chapter 9) support the effectiveness of this group model both in reducing trauma-related symptoms and in addressing such concerns as self-esteem, interpersonal functioning, and affect regulation.

SIMILARITIES AND DIFFERENCES WITH OTHER GROUP MODELS

The TRG has a number of features in common with other models such as those described above. Like these models, the TRG was originally developed for women with complex trauma histories, most commonly childhood physical and/or sexual abuse, and it has subsequently been adapted for other populations (see Chapter 8). Like most other group treatment models, the TRG is a time-limited therapy with weekly 90-minute group meetings. In this treatment guide, we recommend a 16-week format, but this is a flexible aspect of the group design. This duration is similar to many other groups (e.g., Bradley & Follingstad, 2003; Chard, 2005; Lubin & Johnson, 2008), although models range from a minimum of 10 weeks (Alexander, Neimeyer, Mack, & Harter, 1989) to a maximum of 1 year (Harris, 1998). Like most other group models we have reviewed, the TRG is not designed to be a standalone treatment; rather, it is intended to complement and enhance individual psychotherapy.

The TRG differs from most existing group treatment models for survivors of interpersonal trauma in a number of important ways.

1. Unlike the TRG, most other group models appear most suitable for survivors in early recovery. Some authors make this predisposition explicit: For example, the focus of SS is on making small changes in the present, and exploration of the past is explicitly ruled out. Similarly, TREM is designed for women "who live on the social, emotional or economic margin" (Harris, 1998, pp. xi–xii), focusing on topics related to present-day survival and using a question-and-answer format. Wolfsdorf and Zlotnick (2001) invoke the concept of recovery stages and state that the focus of their group is "stabilization." Exceptions include

TCGP, which could be characterized as a "hybrid" model, and cognitive processing therapy for sexual abuse survivors (CPT-SA; Chard, 2005), which utilizes exposure and is not based on a theoretical model of stage-based treatment. There are thus relatively few manualized group treatments available for survivors who have established some safety and stability and are ready to do "Stage 2" trauma work.

2. Reflecting its Stage 2 focus, the TRG approach differs in format from most other groups. Other manualized group treatments are more didactic, with the therapist in the role of educator and a different topic selected for discussion each week. Some other groups include lectures by the therapist (e.g., Lubin & Johnson, 2008; Wolfsdorf & Zlotnick, 2001), handouts with a question-and-answer format (Najavits, 2002), a blackboard (Harris, 1998), or homework (Chard, 2005; Lubin & Johnson, 2008).

In contrast, the format for the TRG is co-created by the group members and the therapists. The organizing principle is the task assigned to each group member, namely, to define and then to achieve a personal goal related to the trauma. There is no set agenda or topic for each meeting; rather, the structure is negotiated through the ritual of taking time. Each group member claims time—first, to share a meaningful part of her story, and then to receive feedback from the other group members. The group leaders serve as timekeepers, taking responsibility for ensuring that time will be shared equally and fairly.

3. The TRG differs from other group models by explicitly developing the therapeutic potential of group interaction. In the TRG model, the interactions of group members are the source of healing and empowerment. In bearing witness to one another's stories, and in supporting one another's efforts to define and achieve a goal, group members discover that they are capable of giving and receiving compassion and care. We believe that trauma survivors, who so often lack self-empathy, may first experience empathy for other survivors and only later allow themselves the experience of being seen and heard in the group. The group leaders' role is to facilitate the development of these empathic capacities. In the ritual of giving and receiving feedback, the group leaders establish a frame within which group members can experience acceptance, belonging and mutuality. This manual offers group leaders specific instruction in techniques for containing potentially disruptive and negative group interactions and for modeling and encouraging accurate empathic feedback.

In many other models, the rationale for a group modality is weak. The SS model, for example, can be implemented either as an individual or a group treatment. Cost-effectiveness is the only rationale offered for a group. Similarly, Ryan, Nitsun, Gilbert, and Mason (2005) offered their clients a choice of the same 12-week treatment module in either an individual or group format. No attention was given to the ways in which the group therapy experience might differ from individual treatment. Not surprisingly, their data showed no differences in effectiveness between the two formats. The TREM manual, which offers extensive instruction on the content to be covered, offers no specific instructions on how to create a safe and supportive group environment. In our view, the heavily didactic structure of most trauma survivor groups militates against the development of strong bonds among group members.

The group that most closely resembles our model in this respect is the 16-week TCGP. The authors state that the objective of the model is "to utilize the power of group dynamics to penetrate the maladaptive patterns of trauma victims" (Lubin & Johnson, 2008, p. 3). They offer some examples of group members giving one another positive feedback, and they clearly intend for the group to become a witnessing community that can correct one another's "faulty cognitions" about the trauma. However, they do not offer any specific technical advice about how to foster these positive interactions, nor how to handle conflict or potential areas of conflict, such as time sharing.

4. The concept of empowerment is key to the TRG, which was developed from an explicitly feminist understanding of the social basis of gender-based violence and sexual exploitation. While this feature is shared with TREM (Harris, 1998), it is absent from most other group models, where instead the focus on women is explained simply by referencing the high prevalence of sexual abuse in the general population and the resulting psychological disturbances that so often lead women survivors to seek treatment. In these other treatments, the absence of a feminist analysis is sometimes evident in the way the issues of gender-based violence are explained. For example, the fifth session in TCGP is titled "Womanhood: My Ally or My Enemy?" Women in this session are informed that men as well as women can be victims of sexual abuse and instructed that "raping and molestation have nothing to do with your gender" but should be seen simply as an abuse of power by an individual perpetrator (Lubin & Johnson, 2008, p. 61).

We believe, on the contrary, that raping and molestation have a great deal to do with gender and that an explicitly feminist social analysis is essential to the understanding of gender-based violence. We understand violence against women both as an expression of male social dominance and as a means of perpetuating it through terror and humiliation. Without this basic framework, survivors have no way to make sense of their intense emotional reactions to the "little rapes," the ordinary humiliations and dangers of women's daily lives. A similar set of power dynamics apply when men and boys are victimized, most commonly by other men. As in the case of violence against women, perpetrators seek to dominate and humiliate their victims; in this case, however, male victims frequently equate their humiliated state with a feminized gender identity. To be subordinated is to be deprived of manhood, to be made into a "sissy" or a "bitch," that is, to be made a woman. This social understanding is particularly apt when the TRG is adapted for male trauma survivors.

CONCLUSION

In this chapter, we contextualized the TRG as a group founded on a feminist analysis of gender-based interpersonal violence and reflecting a stage-based approach to recovery from interpersonal violence. We described the prevalence and impact of interpersonal violence. We reviewed the literature on individual and group treatments for complex PTSD and argued that the TRG is unique in its design and clear focus on treating survivors who are in the second stage of recovery from interpersonal violence. The next chapter provides an in-depth description of the core features of the TRG and its structure and format before we proceed to discuss the "nuts and bolts" of its implementation.

CHAPTER 2

Overview of
the Trauma Recovery Group

THEORETICAL INFLUENCES ON THE TRG

As we noted in Chapter 1, the TRG is based on a feminist analysis of interpersonal violence and a stage-based model of trauma recovery. In regard to its theoretical orientation, the TRG integrates various treatment approaches but is most strongly influenced by psychodynamic and cognitive-behavioral traditions. The development of the TRG was informed by James Mann's (1973/1996, p. 74) psychoanalytically based model of time-limited psychotherapy, which was "designed to take advantage of, to utilize constructively in the service of the patient, the element of time that . . . is so steadfastly avoided in the mental lives of both patients and therapists." The TRG is insight-oriented in its emphasis on the value of making conscious connections between past experiences (particularly past trauma) and present behavior. The group is based on a psychodynamic understanding of self in relation. The TRG recognizes the impact of early experiences and relationships with caregivers in shaping individuals' development and expectations of self and others. It assumes that "individuals repeat emotional and behavioral patterns that were of value to them when they attempted to solve difficulties in the past. . . . Interactions in the interpersonal field of a group often evoke these repetitious patterns, which are the essence of transference" (Rutan, Stone, & Shay, 2007, p. 81). Through exposure to a myriad of possible interactions, group psychotherapy provides unparalleled opportunities for "working through" these interpersonal patterns. In the TRG, this "working through" is focused on patterns and behaviors relevant to the member's trauma-related goal.

The TRG also incorporates several important aspects of CBT. The ultimate purpose of treatment is to effect behavioral change in the present in a domain of functioning that has been impacted by trauma. It also shares with CBT an emphasis on setting and tracking concrete and achievable goals. In its focus on retelling aspects of the trauma, the model recognizes the role of exposure and habituation in reducing the emotional valence of traumatic memories. Where faulty beliefs related to the experience of trauma are identified in the retelling, these are respectfully and empathically challenged by group members and leaders. Group leaders provide psychoeducation when appropriate, which is another feature shared with CBT approaches. Using Foy et al.'s (2001) formulation, detailed in the preceding chapter, the TRG can thus best be described as an "uncovering" rather than a "covering" approach to group trauma treatment.

GENERAL GOALS

The TRG has a number of overriding goals that resemble Yalom and Leszcz's (2005) description of curative factors in group therapy (but which are particularly salient for trauma survivors at the second stage of recovery) in addressing the negative impact of trauma on perceptions of self and others, an effect that frequently endures even after safety is established and symptoms have stabilized. The accomplishment of these general goals both facilitates and is promoted by participants' work on their individualized goals, which are described later in this chapter.

Relieving Shame

Shame is one of the enduring effects of chronic interpersonal trauma. Fonagy, Target, Gergely, Allen, and Bateman (2003, p. 445) describe the shame of the abused child as "an intense and destructive sense of self-disgust, verging on self-hatred." Participating in a group with fellow survivors can provide a powerful antidote to the shame and stigma often associated with traumas such as sexual abuse and domestic violence. The simple process of relating one's story in a safe and structured setting and recognizing one's commonalities with others who have been traumatized can be a tremendous relief for survivors who have borne the burden of silence for many years. Experiencing the acceptance of group members who have heard the survivor's story counteracts this impaired self-reference. The feminist orientation of the group also expands the reference frame for understanding experiences of violation from one of personal responsibility to one recognizing the broader societal problem.

Reducing Isolation

After experiencing trauma, it is common for survivors to feel an overwhelming sense of being alone and disconnected from others. Feelings of shame, trust difficulties, and trauma-related symptoms can all contribute to social withdrawal and impairments in interpersonal functioning. The experience of connecting with other group members who have had similar experiences and difficulties is a powerful vehicle for combating these feelings of isolation as well as laying a foundation for enabling the survivor to connect or reconnect with safe others in their outside lives, which is one of the ultimate goals of the recovery process.

Promoting Mastery

Extreme feelings of helplessness are frequently a core component of the experience of trauma. Prolonged and repeated trauma can result in a pervasive sense of powerlessness, a phenomenon known in the psychological literature as "learned helplessness" (Seligman, 1972) and associated with depression and other ill effects on mental health. Furthermore, survivors often come to treatment with low self-esteem and a limited sense of personal agency. Through the process of choosing, pursuing, and then achieving a goal, group members discover that their intentions and actions can effectuate change. The mastery experience that the group celebrates is a powerful antidote to the feelings of helplessness attendant to victimization. It is for this reason that a lot of time and care is taken in defining a suitable goal, one that is both psychologically meaningful and realistically achievable. It has been our observation that, regardless of the nature of the individual goal pursued by members, the experience of doing so successfully promotes fundamental shifts in their sense of control and self-efficacy. It is hoped that survivors will leave the group not only with a sense of pride derived from this particular accomplishment but also with the skills and confidence to set and accomplish goals in other areas of their lives.

Promoting Empowerment

As noted in Chapter 1, the feminist vision of empowerment is a guiding philosophical underpinning of the TRG. The group promotes empowerment in a number of ways:

1. It brings survivors out of isolation and into connection with one another.
2. It counters the enforced passivity of social subordination with the psychological experiences of initiative and agency involved in accomplishing a goal.
3. It provides members with choice and control over the content of their therapeutic work.
4. It structures interactions in a way that conveys the notion that everyone is equal and deserves to be heard.
5. It gives the member opportunities to contribute to the goal accomplishment and healing of other survivors.
6. By providing a social and ecological analysis of interpersonal violence (Harvey, 1996), the group assists members in enlarging their understanding of what has happened to them so that they gain both an emotional and intellectual experience of solidarity.

By taking the initiative to participate in a group of this nature, the client is making a choice to take action on behalf of her own healing.

During the course of the group, participants will frequently evolve from feeling like victims to feeling like survivors. As Herman (1992b) notes in regard to the work of the second stage of recovery:

> Though the survivor is not responsible for the injury that was done to her, she is responsible for her recovery. Paradoxically, acceptance of this apparent injustice is the beginning of empowerment. The only way that the survivor can take full control of her recovery is to take responsibility for it. The only way she can discover her undestroyed strengths is to use them to their fullest. (p. 192)

Modeling Healthy Relationships

As was noted in Chapter 1, disruption in relational capacities is one of the hallmark effects of chronic interpersonal trauma. As Pearlman and Courtois (2005) observe, many symptoms of PTSD are interpersonal in nature (e.g., avoidance of people that trigger recollection of the trauma, feelings of detachment or alienation, irritability). At the same time, these problems make it hard for others to relate to traumatized individuals, compounding their isolation and cutting them off from the social support that has been found to buffer the effects of trauma. These problems are even more complicated for survivors who have experienced severe cumulative trauma and/or were harmed or abandoned by primary care givers or attachment figures. Adult survivors of childhood abuse frequently experience sensitivity to rejection, abandonment fears, unstable and chaotic relationships, problems in trusting others, and ambivalence regarding intimacy (Briere & Jordan, 2009). Survivor relationships often consist of victim–perpetrator bonds and dynamics that may be expressed in repeated abusive relationships and high rates of revictimization (Cloitre et al., 2006).

Safe attachment has been identified as an important indicator of recovery status among abuse survivors (Tummala-Narra, Liang, & Harvey, 2007). The highly structured format for peer interaction in the group allows for individuals to form safe connections and attachments with one another that are based on mutual support and reciprocity. Furthermore, the co-leaders, in their interactions with each other and with group members, provide an experience of caring and respectful authority figures collaborating to promote the safety and growth of all participants. In this way, the group experience is designed to provide an alternative "template" that can be used by members to identify and cultivate safe and mutually supportive relationships outside of the group.

Integrating Past and Present, Memory and Affect

Courtois et al. (2009) describe the primary accomplishment of Stage 2 of recovery as the development of a progressively elaborated and coherent autobiographical narrative based on safe, self-reflective disclosure of traumatic memories and associated reactions. Harvey (1996, p. 12) notes that "in recovery, memory and affect are joined. The past is remembered with feeling. Cognitive recollections of traumatic events include some remembrance and incorporate some re-experiencing of the affects and bodily states that initially accompanied those events." She adds that memories are also interwoven with new feelings born of remembering and reflecting on the past. In the TRG, the focus on a goal that is related to each client's trauma history and relevant to her present life provides a context for disclosure and making connections between past and present. Integration of memory and affect is promoted as members gradually share relevant traumatic memories, and they are assisted by the group leaders and other members in noticing and differentiating feelings associated both with remembering these experiences and sharing them in the group. Where necessary, group leaders intervene either to deepen the connection between memory and affect or to promote affective modulation so that the client's information-processing capacity is preserved. Group leaders also help members to integrate the feedback they receive from the group into their stories, often resulting in dramatic shifts in members' understanding of their experiences. Techniques for facilitating such integration are examined and exemplified in Chapters 4–6, which cover the implementation of the TRG approach.

Providing a Future Orientation

One of the hallmark effects of psychological trauma is a foreshortened sense of the future. Survivors are frequently preoccupied by past events and may feel hopeless about the possibility of change. The act of planning a goal and taking action toward that goal can be extremely helpful in fostering a newfound sense of hope for the future. Also, because survivors are often at different points even within this second stage of recovery, participating in a group with others who may be earlier or further along in the recovery process can promote both a sense of accomplishment and hopefulness for what lies ahead.

KEY ELEMENTS

The TRG has six key elements that define its structure and make it unique relative to other group models. The TRG is *trauma-focused*. It is *time-limited* and *goal-oriented*. It is structured by the technique of *time sharing*, which ensures equal participation. Its *process is supportive*, with emphasis on learning to give and receive empathic feedback. Finally, we strongly recommend *co-leadership* of the group as the ideal model, with the understanding that many circumstances may make this ideal impossible to realize. These basic characteristics are described in detail below.

Focus on Trauma

As a Stage 2 group, the TRG is trauma-focused in that it involves the exploration and processing of relevant traumatic memories as members work on their present-oriented goals. As Herman (1992b) notes, work at this stage of recovery involves reconstructing the story, transforming traumatic memories, and mourning losses associated with the trauma. During the early sessions of the group, members tell the group their story as a means of contextualizing their goal and its relation to their trauma. In doing so, participants also place their trauma in the context of their life and developmental history. In this process, it is not uncommon for members to broaden their perspective on the aspects of their history that they perceive as contributing to their current difficulties. For example, a member who came to the group reporting a history of physically abusive adult relationships realized how her family environment of emotional neglect and verbal abuse predisposed her to becoming involved in violent relationships in her teen years. She understood for the first time that she longed for attention and was not able to heed the warning signs that her partners would become physically violent, as she was so accustomed to the verbal abuse that preceded the physical violence.

For some clients, transformation of a traumatic memory may be the explicit goal of their group participation, for example, in the case of a survivor who indicated that she wants to be able to recall her abuse experience without experiencing a primary reaction of shame and self-blame. This client delayed the telling of the narrative, taking time to develop trust and to let herself and the group know what meaningful support might look like in response to her disclosure. She also made sure that she had several weeks after the telling to experience herself as part of a group that knew what happened and expressed respect and caring for her. This powerful experience of safe self-disclosure in the supportive relational context of the group environment had the power to enable her to transform her own self-loathing and shame. For others, transformation of memory may be incidental to their goal but also nonetheless an important aspect of their group participation. Members are most helpful in supporting one another deal with present-day issues if they understand what happened in the past. For example, a participant who worried that the perpetrator might abuse other young family members and wanted guidance on what to do now was asked about her past abuse experiences. What happened? Did she think anyone knew? If she told no adults, was it because she feared no one would believe her, and did she fear that would happen now with her young relative? Did she worry that the child would be further hurt by disclosure, and, if so, what steps could she take to prevent unnecessary harm? Looking back now as an adult, who might she have enlisted as a potential ally?

Another aspect of sharing the trauma narrative has to do with members who have already disclosed their story to family members and realize in the group that they did so without sharing any details of what happened to them or what the impact has been on them as adults (Schatzow & Herman, 1989). Although this more detailed disclosure may be met with a reaction similar to the original one, it creates a real opportunity for the survivor to give voice to the experience and hand the shame back to the perpetrators and bystanders. This type of disclosure can be enormously empowering so long as the client is not looking for acknowledgment but rather a chance to speak her truth. The goal for this member could be to prepare for this event, determining the best process for accomplishing it (e.g., a meeting in her therapist's office, a letter, or a phone call) and clarifying what she wants to say. It would be ideal if this event occurred over the course of the group sessions, but even if this were not possible, planning for such an event would be a very worthy goal. This type of work would not be possible in a Stage 1 group (where safety and self-care are not yet firmly established) because the process described above can be destabilizing for clients in early recovery.

Although formalized exposure procedures are not part of this group model, exposure and habituation take place as members revisit their trauma histories and retell their stories either as a means of contextualizing their goals or as part of their goal work. Group leaders assist members in working within the "therapeutic window" (Briere, 1996) in the ways we describe in subsequent chapters so that they are connected with affect but not overwhelmed by it. Questions asked and observations offered by group leaders and members facilitate the integration of thoughts and feelings associated with the trauma. We do not view exposure as sufficient in transforming the distortions in perceptions of self and others experienced by survivors of chronic and prolonged interpersonal trauma. In this regard, the experience of retelling the trauma story or parts of it in the relational context of the group is crucial. In response to the caring and empathetic feedback from other members who "bear witness" to the member's story, the client's negative views of herself are challenged and ultimately give way to a more compassionate stance toward her own behavior and increased self-worth. Expectations that others in the wider community will be disapproving or abusive are also countered by the respectful and supportive reactions of group members. When such support is offered by respected group members with whom the client identifies and who have made themselves equally vulnerable within the group, this "corrective" feedback is much harder to dismiss than when it is provided by the client's individual therapist or the group leader. The individual therapist may be regarded as someone who is well meaning but could be "lying" about the supportive feedback because he or she just wants the client to feel better. In addition to receiving compassionate responses to her own story, each group member feels compassion for others. Often it is the authenticity of her own deeply felt experience that convinces a group member of the genuineness of others' compassion.

The third major task of the second stage of recovery involves mourning the losses associated with the trauma. As Herman (1992b) notes, coming to terms with these losses can be an extremely difficult and painful process. These losses may involve actual physical integrity as well as "internal psychological structures of a self securely attached to others" (p. 188). In addition, clients frequently mourn the loss of "possible futures" as they reflect on the ways in which their lives might have been different had the trauma not occurred. In the supportive context of the TRG, members inevitably grieve painful losses related to their histories. With the help of the group leaders where needed, the group is challenged to allow this grieving to occur without prematurely intervening to shut it down. Other members are usually an important source of encouragement and inspiration to clients in the midst of grieving, reminding them that grief does not last forever and that acknowledging and processing losses is an essential step before one can move on with life. This is a key component because many trauma survivors believe that effective coping means *never* mourning the losses. A common fear is "If I were to allow myself to feel the sadness, I would never, ever stop crying."

An important aspect of this mourning process frequently involves taking responsibility for behaviors and choices that the survivor ultimately regrets as well as finding ways to "put things right" in the present whenever possible. For example, Anna's group goal involved preparing herself to attend her son's college graduation. Anna reported a strained and distant relationship with her son, based on her guilt at not having protected him adequately from his violent father and her awareness that he was angry toward her for this neglect. In preparing herself emotionally for this event, Anna expressed a lot of remorse for not being more protective. The group listened empathetically to her tearful confessions about the ways in which she perceived herself as having failed him. In the feedback, members who had themselves had a nonprotective parent appreciated the step that Anna had taken in assuming responsibility for her behavior, something their parents had never done. Group members also noted how Anna's real fear for her own safety had kept her paralyzed. Anna decided that she wanted to have a conversation with her son prior to his graduation expressing her feelings about not having intervened sufficiently and letting him know that she wanted to play a more active and supportive role in his life going forward if he were willing. Anna used her group time to rehearse what she would say and anticipate possible reactions from her son. Toward the end of the group sessions and prior to his graduation, Anna spoke with him. Although he continued to express hurt and anger, he also indicated that he was willing to work on improving their relationship. Anna concluded her time in group treatment saying that she felt more compassionate toward herself and more hopeful about the future of her relationship with her son.

Time Limit

The TRG is not an open-ended psychotherapy group but rather one deliberately designed to provide clients with a limited amount of time to accomplish their goals. This time limit encourages trauma survivors to engage in emotionally intense work that might not be possible for them in a more open-ended format. It also helps preserve the focus on goals as opposed to interpersonal process. Although we do not claim that all the work of recovery is completed within the time limit, we are teaching group members an important recovery skill: they learn that they can accomplish a piece of work by focusing in on a specific behavioral outcome and that this approach can be applied to other goals of recovery. Not everything has to be done at once. It is possible for a client to repeat the TRG group with a different goal. However, we generally recommend that clients take a break between groups in order to consolidate what they have achieved and have time to practice applying it in their daily lives.

Goal Orientation

A key component of the TRG is the selection by each client of a personally meaningful goal that is related to her trauma history and its present consequences. Individualized goals allow for specificity in tackling what each group member feels is particularly challenging about her trauma history. Given the range of tasks that survivors may face in this mid-stage of recovery, it makes sense to employ a model that allows each member to achieve mastery over the issue that she finds most salient. For some clients, this goal relates to residual trauma-related symptoms; for others, it pertains to the impact of trauma on their sense of self, relationships, or ability to participate in the wider world. As has been noted, the purpose of the individual goal is both to provide a structure and focus for the client's group participation and to promote a sense of mastery and self-efficacy. The process of defining a goal begins in the initial intake interview and continues through the early stages of the group. Once the group member has defined a goal, the group tracks her progress, helps her to redefine her goal if necessary, and celebrates her success. During the concluding phase, members take stock of what they have achieved relative to their goals and consider their next therapeutic steps in light of their accomplishments.

The client's goal also provides a starting point and organizing framework for disclosing her trauma history and processing salient memories. During the early stage of the group treatment once goals have been identified, members talk about how those goals came to be important in their life. This process inevitably involves reviewing aspects of their trauma history and honing in on particular memories that were most influential. For some members, detailed retelling *is* their goal work—for example, in the case of a member who wants to be able to remain present in her body while recalling the trauma, or one who is preparing to disclose to a family member or significant other that she is an incest survivor. For others, retelling is undertaken with the purpose of separating fears and assumptions from the past from the reality of present situations relevant to their identified goals so that they are empowered to make choices rather than replay old trauma-based scripts.

When thinking about how to help members formulate useful goals, the leaders should be thinking about the particular tasks that members of their targeted population are facing. How might these tasks be accomplished in small steps? What are the psychological, socio-economic, and political impediments to achieving these tasks? The process of taking large recovery issues, analyzing them, and breaking them down into concrete achievable goals may be a new skill for some therapists. Several guidelines for assisting clients in arriving at the goals that are most beneficial in counteracting the effects of trauma and promoting healing are detailed below:

- *The goal should be trauma-related.* Although this statement may sound self-evident given the nature of the group, it is important that all clients work on goals that are in some way related to their trauma history. While many clients may be simultaneously dealing with problems that are clearly not related to their histories of trauma, these should not be the focus of their work in the group.

- *The goal should be present-oriented.* Goals should relate to the impact of the client's trauma history on relevant aspects of her present functioning. It is important to explore which areas of her life continue to be affected by the trauma. Once she has identified some core areas, a common theme may emerge that can be honed into a goal for the group treatment. Alternatively, a particular area may stand out as most pressing in regard to the need for intervention.

- *The goal should be realistic and achievable.* Goals should be realistically achievable within the time span of the group treatment. If a goal seems too large or overly ambitious, it is crucial to reassess and modify it so that the client can ultimately experience a sense of mastery. For example, a client whose symptoms have interfered with her ability to maintain employment may come with a goal of getting back to work in her chosen profession. Apart from any practical considerations involved in finding a suitable job, for someone who has not worked for some time it may be more realistic to start by finding and maintaining a volunteer job several hours per week. The client could use her group time to reflect on some of the challenges she confronts in doing so and how these relate to her trauma memories, and work on overcoming them as a step toward seeking paid employment.

- *The goal should be concrete.* It is important that the goal be adequately detailed and concretely defined that the client is able to recognize when it has been accomplished or how much progress she has made in doing so. The more measurable the goal, the better. For example, many clients come to the group with the somewhat vague goal of "feeling better about myself." For a particular client, this goal may be operationalized as "taking better care of myself," which may then be further developed and made more substantive as "engaging in at least one self-care activity each day." The client's group time could be spent reflecting on her reactions to engaging in self-care and the obstacles to doing so.

- *The goal should be specific.* Many clients come to the group with a goal that is overly broad. It is the task of the group leaders to help the client specify it sufficiently so that it can be accomplished while still retaining its significance to the client. For example, a client may enter the group with general goal of wanting to feel less isolated, whereupon this goal may be usefully recast as joining one or more social groups.

- *The goal setting should be collaborative.* While goals should be personally relevant and ultimately originate with the client, developing and refining the goals should be a collaborative process that is part of the work of the group. Although it is beneficial for clients to have some sense of a potential goal at the start of the group, it is expected that their goal may be transformed during the first few sessions. Even when one comes to the group with a relatively clear and well-defined goal, it is helpful to receive and incorporate feedback from the group leaders and the other members before committing oneself to its precise expression. It is also helpful for clients to share in developing their goal with their individual therapist to gain additional feedback from a person who is likely to have a more extensive knowledge of their history and abilities.

- *Goals can be renegotiated.* Members' goals are not "set in stone" for the duration of the group sessions; indeed, they often evolve over time as it becomes clearer what is and is not achievable during the time frame of the group. For example, a client may begin the group therapy with the goal of confronting a nonprotective parent. Over the course of the group sessions, she may decide that she is not emotionally ready to do so and may choose instead to have a conversation about her abuse with a sibling. Less frequently, after a few sessions a member may find that she has achieved her goal (e.g., telling the group about an episode of abuse without dissociating); in this case, she may choose to extend her goal, for example, to disclosing the abuse to her significant other in a connected way. Renegotiation of goals should be treated as an integral part of the therapeutic process so as to promote a sense of mastery and success and to discourage feelings of shame and failure.

- *Clients may have in-group or out-of-group goals.* Some clients select in-group goals that involve working directly on their goal during their group time. These goals often involve disclosing a piece of the trauma narrative with affect and remaining present in the group while doing so. It is important that this retelling have relevance to a present-day difficulty. Alternatively, a client who struggles with trust difficulties related to her trauma may choose to work on the goal of allowing other members to know her better over the course of the therapy. Her work may involve sharing aspects of herself that she usually conceals and reflecting on her experience of doing so in the interpersonal context of the group. Other clients may work on out-of-group goals. For example, a client who experiences anxiety in social interactions with men may seek out such situations incrementally and use her group time to explore further her emotional and cognitive reactions and their connections to her trauma history. Alternatively, a group member may choose the goal of disclosing her abuse to members of her family and may use her group time to prepare herself for this disclosure. It has been our experience that out-of-group goals are generally easier to plan, recognize, and report back on, with attendant celebratory feedback. In considering the group as a whole, generally we recommend that members have a mix of in-group and out-of-group goals. When all or most members focus on in-group goals, this emphasis can create too much interpersonal intensity. It may also contribute to a feeling of not having sufficient time, since members' work is centered around what they are doing in the group rather than what other steps they may be taking outside the group.

The following illustration is offered of how a client's goal is first identified, refined, and then pursued over the course of the therapy. In the screening interview, "Cathy" stated that she would like her goal for the group to involve becoming less isolated. The group leaders encouraged her to think about ways to make this goal more specific and break it down into concrete steps in order to identify something that could be accomplished within the time frame of a 4-month treatment. At the start of the group, Cathy indicated that she had been talking about this goal with her therapist and had realized that she found it difficult to pursue new relationships because she worried about being perceived as needy or flawed. A group leader asked if there was anyone in her current life who she would like to know better, and she reported that there was someone at work who might be a potential friend, as they shared common interests. Her goal evolved into being able to ask her coworker to join her for lunch or coffee. In preparing to take this step, during the group's earliest sessions Cathy used some of her time to speak about her fears of being judged and their origin in her childhood environment, which was characterized by physical and verbal abuse. During succeeding sessions, Cathy described her experience of having been repeatedly humiliated by her father and brothers (and later by peers at school) when she made her needs and wishes known. She recalled painful feelings of shame associated with these experiences and reflected on how they ultimately led her to avoid initiating interpersonal relationships. Through empathic questioning and comments from group members, Cathy was able to recognize the ways in which her fears had kept her removed from the feedback that might normally counter the negative messages she had received in childhood. She was also reminded that she had no reason to expect that this particular coworker would reject her. Strengthened by this new perspective on her behavior and its consequences and encouraged by the acceptance she experienced from the group, Cathy indicated a readiness to act on her goal. Group members shared examples of ways in which they had approached people that they had wanted to know better, helping Cathy decide how to approach her coworker. She also used her group time to speak about how she would manage feelings of disappointment if the advance were rebuffed and how, in reaching out, she would consider the goal accomplished irrespective of the recipient's response. Cathy approached her coworker and suggested that they meet for coffee one day after work. Her coworker responded positively, they met, and Cathy felt that they both enjoyed the interaction. The following week, her coworker invited her to see a movie together. During the next group session, Cathy shared these developments with the group, inciting both applause and other positive reinforcement. She was asked to reflect on the impact of this experience on her beliefs about others' negative perceptions about herself.

Time Sharing

During each session, usually about three members volunteer to work on their respective goals, and each member's "turn" is divided between sharing their perspectives and receiving feedback from others. This time-sharing approach enables members to work on their various goals without having to actively compete for time. It ensures that no single person will dominate the group, nor will anyone be overlooked or allowed to avoid participating. With its insistence on equal time sharing, the group models a community based on equal participation. This approach facilitates moving from the work of one person to the next. Dividing time between sharing and feedback recognizes the importance of reciprocity, empathy, and mutuality in relationships, concepts that are emphasized in feminist psychology (Surrey, Stiver, Miller, Kaplan, & Jordan, 1991). In taking responsibility for time keeping, the group leaders remove one of the most potentially contentious group process issues from the arena of conflict. How specifically to implement time sharing is described later (in the section on "Individual Session Format"). It is important to note here that, unlike the situation in process-oriented psychotherapy groups, structured time sharing requires that group leaders assume a very active and directive role in managing time and controlling group interactions. Co-leaders have to interrupt members to let them know when it is time to shift from sharing to feedback and when a member's "turn" is almost done. Especially during the early stages of the therapy, when members are becoming oriented to the group's procedures, leaders also sometimes need to intervene when a member strays off the topic or gives inappropriate feedback. Technical considerations in doing so are reviewed in Chapters 4–6 of this volume, on implementation of TRG therapy.

Supportive Process

Therapy groups for trauma survivors in the second stage of recovery generally manifest high cohesion and low conflict tolerance among members (Herman, 1992b). The TRG is intentionally structured to create an atmosphere of mutual support and interpersonal safety as members work on their goals. These supportive connections both sustain the member while she processes painful material from the past and also provide her with a new relational experience of safe attachment. This favorable environment is fostered in several ways. As noted above, providing for time sharing means that members do not have to actively vie for time within the group. Allocating a portion of time to the process of receiving feedback means that members who have volunteered to share in a session also have the experience of others attending and responding to them. They hear other members identifying with their experiences, offering empathy and compassion, expressing respectful curiosity, and sharing suggestions. This group model requires that members be attentive and engaged in the group even when it is not their turn to share. The group leaders model thoughtful and supportive feedback by making observations about what the member has shared and asking relevant questions, encouraging group members to do the same and thereby become active agents in one another's recovery. If a member is particularly withdrawn or dissociated, group leaders should notice and gently intervene to assist her in becoming more present and engaged by exploring with her what might help to facilitate her participation. Group leaders also check in with members often on how they are receiving the feedback that has been offered. If feedback is offered or heard with a critical tone, group leaders will intervene quickly to provide the speaker with an opportunity to reword her thoughts or reframe what she has said. Group leaders will also take careful note of how a member is responding to *positive* feedback, as this is often hard to take in fully. If needed, the leaders may deliberately slow down this process to help the member identify what gets in the way of internalizing feedback and find ways of making herself more receptive to listeners' feedback. For example, they may ask the sharing member what she is thinking or notices feeling in her body as she hears the feedback. If it appears that there are distortions in her understanding of the feedback, the group members providing it may be asked to reword what they have said or clarify their intentions and meaning.

As in any group situation, group members may feel a variety of negative feelings toward one another such as anger, dislike, and envy and competition based both on real interactions in the present group situation and projections from past relationships. Similarly, interpersonal conflicts are bound to arise. In process-oriented psychotherapy groups, the exploration of such reactions and conflicts is usually encouraged and ultimately facilitates members' "working through" the interpersonal problems that brought them to the group. In the TRG, these reactions and conflicts are typically *not* explored—for two reasons: (1) to maintain the focus on members' individual goals and (2) to preserve interpersonal safety and cohesiveness in the time-limited group. Usually, when such situations arise, the co-leaders may intervene by acknowledging the feelings or conflict being expressed and explaining that these feelings should be explored further in members' individual therapy (for the reasons mentioned above). An exception may be made when a process issue is clearly relevant to a member's individualized goal. In this case, group leaders may frame the situation as an opportunity for the member to take steps toward her goal, either through increased understanding of self and other or through trying out a new interpersonal behavior. The example of Kate and Rose, below, may help to differentiate how interpersonal conflict is dealt with in the TRG as compared with a process-oriented group.

In her therapy group, Kate gives other members a lot of advice while sharing little of her own vulnerability. After this pattern occurred numerous times, Rose had an outburst of frustration, accusing Kate of "acting like you're better than all of us." What should the group leaders do? The answer depends on the kind of group involved. In a process-oriented group, this kind of confrontation may present an opportunity for Kate to explore her feelings about being criticized in this manner, the ways in which her behavior may contribute to this perception, and the purpose that it serves. Rose might explore her feelings of anger and shame at Kate's perceived condescension and how this reaction relates to the interpersonal conflicts she experiences outside the group. The group leader would also likely elicit other group members' reactions to this situation if these were not readily expressed.

In contrast, in the TRG, the group leaders would intervene quickly to deescalate conflict and try to repair group cohesion. After briefly checking in with Kate about how she is feeling, the leaders would acknowledge that members may be having a variety of emotional reactions to the interpersonal conflict, reiterate the importance of mutual respect, and perhaps offer some psychoeducational comments about different interpersonal styles that members bring to a group. They might then provide Rose an opportunity to reword her feedback in a way that could be more helpful to Kate. If the interpersonal conflict is not relevant to the goals of either Kate or Rose, the group leaders would likely point to the goal focus and time limit of the group and encourage Kate and Rose to process their feelings further in individual therapy. In the rare case where this solution might not be sufficient, the group leaders could also meet with Kate and/or Rose outside of session (the group will always be informed of such a meeting) to help them find a way to manage their reactions sufficiently well to them to continue to participate in the group. These interventions would not occur in a process group, where there is an emphasis on keeping group interactions and process in the group.

If it were determined that the conflict was relevant to Kate's and/or Rose's goals, the leaders would solicit their agreement to continue processing this interaction during the member's respective turn. However, the processing would focus on the aspects of the interaction directly relevant to each one's goal rather than involve open-ended exploration about members' feelings about the conflict. For instance, if Rose's goal in group was to respond less reactively to certain interpersonal triggers, during her turn her reaction in this situation and its impact on Kate and the group could be explored, and Rose could be helped to identify more appropriate ways of managing and expressing her frustration. Similarly, if Kate's goal involved allowing herself to feel "known" by the group by sharing her feelings associated with her past trauma, her tendency to take on the "co-therapist" role could be understood as a way of avoiding this intimacy. During her turn, her fears of allowing herself to be vulnerable in the group could be explored, and the function of her behavior in keeping others at a distance could be better elucidated and understood. As part of her goal work, Kate might be specifically challenged to "step out of this role and experiment" by allowing herself to be a group member. The group might then be enlisted to help Kate monitor this behavior in a gentle and empathic manner.

Co-leadership

Co-leadership (i.e., two leaders conducting the group together) serves a number of specific purposes in the TRG. For the group members, effective co-leadership sets an example of a relationship of mutuality and collaboration—in contrast to the relationships of domination and subordination that characterize the histories of so many clients. It provides an alternative experience of adult care taking in which power is shared and not abused. It models a cooperative and collective approach to solving problems and handling differences. It minimizes the ready attribution of power and control to a single person. It also communicates the idea that one person cannot "do it all" without support. Co-leadership also has important benefits for the group leaders. The logistics of managing the group from session to session (e.g., contacting others involved in members' care, following up clients who miss sessions) can be shared between two people. Within each session, therapists can share the tasks of attending to the overall group process and tracking individual clients and their goal-related progress. Last but not least, the co-leadership model provides therapists with peer support and feedback that are essential in preventing vicarious traumatization and burnout. Co-leadership is thus highly recommended despite the financial and human resource constraints that can complicate this arrangement.

It is important, however, that group leaders be also aware of the dynamics and complexities involved in co-leadership (for a review, see Delucia-Waack & Fauth, 2004). These dynamics are different for dyads involving dual leadership where one therapist has more experience and power than the other (e.g., in a training situation) versus co-therapy where two leaders are similar in experience and power (Rutan et al., 2007). For trauma survivors in particular, whenever such differences exist, it is crucial that the dynamic of domination and subordination not be reenacted in the leadership pairing (Herman, 1992b). Rutan et al. (2007) note that, irrespective of the specific circumstances of the shared leadership arrangement, several important principles apply: (1) leaders must have fundamental respect for each other, even when considerable differences in experience and skill exist; (2) leaders must allow for sufficient time to explore group process, members' relationships, and their own relationship; and (3) leaders should share a similar theoretical stance.

Having discussed the theoretical underpinnings of the TRG, its overall goals, and its six key features, we now provide an overview of the group. We review the requirements for group leaders and members before describing the details of the group framework and session structure. We conclude by describing some ways in which the work of the group can be reinforced and expanded between sessions.

OVERVIEW OF THE TRG

It is useful to conceptualize the TRG as beginning with a phase of preparation and screening that precedes the group sessions, which in turn unfold over three distinct stages or phases.

Preparation and Screening

Preparation for the TRG entails both establishing logistic arrangements for running the group (e.g., identifying the venue, the preferred time period, and the co-leaders) and ensuring that co-leaders have sufficient familiarity with the treatment model as well as the requisite background and skills to conduct the group properly. A clinical interview with the group leader is considered the primary basis for determining each client's capacity to enter and participate in the psychotherapy group (Rutan et al., 2007). In the TRG, owing to the requirement that safety and stability be established prior to engaging clients in the trauma-focused work of a Stage 2 group as well as the importance of maximizing interpersonal safety in the group, thorough pregroup screening is of utmost importance. The screening process involves a detailed interview that evaluates clients' interest in group therapy, current symptoms, treatment history, coping skills and supports, and risk factors. The co-leaders provide clients with an overview of the group and its purpose and also begin a discussion about possible goals in the event that the client joins the group. With the client's consent, the group leaders also make collateral contacts with any others treating her to assess their support for the client's group participation, providing them with information about the group's structure and function and eliciting their assistance with goal definition. Through these screening procedures, the co-leaders determine whether the group is a good fit with the client's current treatment needs.

Introductory Sessions

The beginning sessions are focused on establishing a sense of safety, structure, and trust within the group as well as formulating individual participants' goals. After initial parameters are established through discussion of the group's purpose, structure, and guidelines, members gradually share information about their lives as they work to provide a context for their individual goals. In this process, members also begin to share their trauma history and its relationship to their goals, initially providing only limited details. Feedback from the group leaders and other members is an integral part of helping clients to define and then refine appropriate goals.

Goal-Work Sessions

As the group becomes more cohesive and members' goals become more clearly defined, the focus normally shifts from providing background context to actively taking steps toward concretely defining the goals that have been identified. As a Stage 2 group, the goal-work stage of the TRG involves some degree of affective sharing of trauma memories in the service of members' goals. Members share their unique traumatic experiences and associated feelings that are related to some ongoing life difficulty or challenge. This phase of the treatment process is charged with strong emotion as members confront painful memories, risk sharing them with others, and begin reaping the benefits of feeling understood and supported by the group. Once these affective and cognitive connections between past and present are made, members may use their group time to try some new behavior, or process more completely something they have done or realized, or reflect on obstacles to doing something that is needed. Feedback may be geared toward supplying support and encouragement, providing a different perspective, and/or making connections that the client had not previously considered. About midway through the treatment, one or more members usually take significant steps toward accomplishing their goals, which provides impetus for others to do likewise.

Concluding Sessions

During the closing sessions, the group reviews the progress that everyone has made in achieving their goals and considers possible next steps and future wishes for each individual. Members reflect on their own progress during the treatment and hopefully they are able to feel a sense of mastery and accomplishment. The leaders provide feedback based on their observations and make recommendations regarding future areas of work for each member.

REQUIREMENTS FOR GROUP LEADERS

Unlike many other groups for trauma survivors, apart from some guidelines for the initial orientation to the group model, the TRG does not have an externally defined curriculum; rather, it is organized around each group member's individual goal work. The group leaders provide structure by taking responsibility for time sharing, ensuring that members' contributions and interactions are directed toward their goals, assisting members in modulating their emotional arousal during trauma processing, monitoring and containing group process, and providing psychoeducation as needed by the group. The specific themes arising in each TRG and the interventions required of leaders will differ, depending on the goals of group members and the specific composition of the group. Owing to this inherent variability, group leaders must be able to draw on a comprehensive understanding of the impact of trauma effects as well as diverse practical skills in working with traumatized clients, as detailed below. Their own access to consultation or supervision, in turn, is a key factor in supporting group leaders' active multifaceted role in successfully implementing TRG therapy.

Relevant Background, Knowledge, and Skills

The leaders of any TRG should be appropriately trained and qualified mental health professionals (e.g., psychologists, social workers, psychiatrists, psychiatric nurses) with experience in working with traumatized clients and facilitating therapy groups. They should be familiar with the clinical literature pertaining to the treatment of adult survivors of childhood abuse and other forms of complex trauma. They should also have a good understanding of group process and treatment. These areas of knowledge and skill are outlined in Table 2.1, with references to key sources containing this information. We suggest that co-leaders review these topics in order to facilitate self-assessment of readiness to conduct the TRG as well as to provide opportunities to acquire or strengthen needed skills. The risks of attempting to run this group without adequate educational background and prior experience include the possibility of retraumatizing members, which may result in compounded pain and the

TABLE 2.1. Required Group Leader Knowledge Base

Topic	Key references
Complex trauma and recovery	
Complex trauma • Characteristics of complex trauma • PTSD, dissociation, and other trauma-related disorders • Impact of trauma on developmental capacities and attachment • Neurobiological consequences of chronic trauma	• Briere & Scott (2006) • Courtois & Ford (2009) • Harvey & Tummala-Narra (2007) • Herman (1992b) • *Journal of Traumatic Stress* (2005) • Wilson, Friedman, & Lindy (2001)

The recovery process
 • Stages of recovery
 • Psychotherapy with trauma survivors
   ▪ Addressing trauma-related symptoms
   ▪ Enhancing affect modulation and interpersonal functioning
   ▪ Countertransference and vicarious traumatization
 • The role of group therapy in the recovery process	

Societal perspectives • Ecological model of trauma and recovery • Sociopolitical roots of interpersonal violence • Multicultural perspectives on trauma and recovery	
Group therapy	
Group therapy basics • Curative factors in group therapy • Stages of group development • Group dynamics • Preparing patients for group therapy • Change process in group psychotherapy	• Bernard & Mackenzie (1994) • Delucia-Waack, Gerrity, Kalodner, & Riva (2004) • Kaplan & Sadock (1994) • Klein & Schermer (2000) • Rutan, Stone, & Shay (2007) • Yalom & Leszcz (2005) • Young & Blake (1999)
Special considerations • Characteristics and types of groups • Special issues in time-limited group therapy • Group therapy with trauma survivors	

likelihood of avoiding future treatment. We strongly urge those considering co-leading a TRG to assess their own readiness objectively and to take sufficient time to acquire the knowledge base and skills we recommend.

The TRG treatment model requires active and responsive co-leaders who intervene readily to promote a sense of safety, maintain the group structure, and model empathetic feedback, particularly during the early stages of the group. Clinicians leading this type of group have to draw on a variety of clinical skills ranging from providing psychoeducation about the impact of trauma, to supporting the development of new interpersonal coping skills, to facilitating the exploration and processing of painful memories. This regimen requires that leaders have the ability to remain flexible and be able to apply whatever interventions are needed during the course of the group sessions. Although significant overlap and integration exist among the functions of the various cognitive-behavioral and dynamically based skills that are employed, a broad overview may help differentiate them, aided by a close review of the case examples provided in the text. In general, such cognitive-behavioral skills as goal setting and tracking, directness in managing time and maintaining focus, containment, and psychoeducation are typically most useful in maintaining the structure of the group, focusing mindfully during periods of individual work, and providing ample opportunities for relevant learning experiences. More dynamically oriented skills are typically utilized to deepen the insights derived from individuals' goal work and include both interpretation and putting one's current behaviors into a developmental perspective. Leaders should also have a repertoire of skills gained from trauma-informed treatments upon which to draw, especially ones that involve modulating affective arousal to an optimal level, including exposure and grounding techniques.

Psychoeducation

Although the TRG is not a psychoeducational group where group leaders have a primarily didactic role, psychoeducational interventions are often indicated in the group and therefore deserve special mention. The use of psychoeducation begins in the screening interview, where group leaders explain the purpose and format of the group and the importance and characteristics of goals. Psychoeducation about group guidelines, structure, and procedures is provided during the early sessions, as described in detail in Chapter 4, and in the concluding phase, described in Chapter 6. In other instances, psychoeducation is provided as the need arises based on members' goal work or experiences in the context of the group. The group leaders therefore need to be able to determine when such a need is present and must be capable of explaining key concepts and processes relevant to trauma and recovery in a brief and comprehensible manner. Psychoeducation may be useful in the following instances: (1) to "depersonalize" a member's experience by putting it in a broader context when she feels alienated and/or different or expresses shame or self-blame; (2) to reinforce a commonality when several group members identify with a particular symptom or experience, especially while cohesion is still building; (3) to minimize or contain group process or conflict that might distract members from their goal-focused work; and (4) to provide a cognitive frame for grounding a member who is overwhelmed by affect. However, leaders should take special care not to use psychoeducation prematurely to shut down affect that might be hard for the group to tolerate but might also be important for a member's goal work.

Psychoeducational input should be both brief and to the point and be used very selectively so as to keep the key focus on members' individual goal work and facilitate their empowerment by making members rather than leaders the central agents in one another's recovery. Psychoeducational comments are usually integrated into the feedback provided by group leaders to individual members, although occasionally (when a psychoeducational issue is salient for many group members and/or addressing it may prevent or diffuse group conflict) group leaders may claim time in the session before or after turn taking to address this issue. Psychoeducational topics that emerge frequently include PTSD, the recovery process, self-care, trust difficulties, anger, shame and guilt, dissociation, the intergenerational impact of trauma, trauma and sexuality, the impact of developmental trauma, and the societal problem of gender-based violence. Table 2.2 lists some frequently occurring psychoeducational topics and directs the reader to examples contained in this treatment guide.

Group leadership skills relevant to short-term groups are also essential and include an awareness of group dynamics and familiarity with techniques for building cohesion and diffusing potential conflict. As already noted, even if they bring different skills to the group, co-leaders should understand the benefits and challenges involved in co-leadership, like and respect each other, and have a shared understanding of trauma and the recovery process. They should also have the willingness and time to collaborate with other treatment professionals (e.g., the client's individual therapist, psychopharmacologist), as this is an important component of this group model (and is also generally good practice).

Because the TRG is a group therapy for survivors of interpersonal violence, issues of power and its possible abuses frequently arise from the outset. Survivors naturally want assurances that the therapist will use power in a benign and constructive manner and will be willing both to witness their trauma stories and to denounce the violence. For example, in a group for survivors of political violence, one could well expect, at a minimum, that the group leaders would have no affiliation with the perpetrator group and preferably that the leaders would have even demonstrated engagement in human rights advocacy. Similarly, in a group for combat veterans, one would naturally expect that the leaders have no affiliation

TABLE 2.2. Common Psychoeducational Topics with Text Examples of Their Use

Topic	Page number(s)
Group structure and process	68–71, 73–75, 77–78, 110–111
Effective feedback/interpersonal skills	77–79, 87–88
Establishing effective interpersonal boundaries	71–72, 111–112
Trauma and self-care	76, 88–89
Differentiating shame and guilt, introducing self-compassion	74–75, 93–94
Confusing being misunderstood with being mistreated	98
Dissociation and grounding	106
Impact of trauma on abilities to trust and form relationships	78, 80–81
Impact of trauma on self-perception	83, 93–94
Sociocultural influences on understanding of trauma and its impact	101
Trauma and sexual responses	94
Impact of trauma on parenting	95

with hostile forces and preferably that they have some firsthand understanding of the soldier's life. In a group for survivors of gender-based violence, the situation is more complex. In general, it would seem preferable for women's groups to be led by women and men's groups to be led by men. However, this arrangement might create a complicated power dynamic—particularly for male survivors, the majority of whom have been abused by men, but also for female survivors who have been abused by women. It is all the more important, therefore, for TRG leaders to understand and be able to communicate their understanding of interpersonal violence as an abuse of power and to anticipate the emotionally fraught reactions that their gender will inevitably inspire. Co-leaders should also be open to exploring and addressing power dynamics within the co-leadership dyad.

In addition to recommending these specific areas of knowledge and skill, we consider it essential that clinicians intending to conduct TRG therapy read this treatment guide thoroughly from start to finish *before* actually organizing such a group. Co-leaders should thoroughly understand the six key elements of the TRG. They should then familiarize themselves with each chapter of this volume so that they have a clear overview of the screening process and each phase of the group process. The flexibility of content in this type of therapy does not lend itself well to a manual that prescribes word for word what clinicians should say. This treatment guide includes many verbatim examples of group leaders' explanations and interventions, but these are offered as examples only; clinicians new to the model are encouraged to find their own words as they assume the leadership role. We strongly advise group leaders not to bring the treatment guide into sessions or read from it verbatim, as this is disruptive to the development of the relational connections among participants that the group strives to foster. For the same reasons, group leaders are discouraged from taking notes during sessions. However, it is well worth the effort to take detailed notes following each session, recording the progress in each member's goal work as well as important group process developments.

Supervision

Regardless of their level of expertise, group leaders must have regular access to supervision or consultation with a clinician who is experienced in conducting and supervising trauma treatment and group therapy, is familiar with this treatment approach, and has read the manual thoroughly. Supervision is an *essential* component of all clinical work, since it both assists clinicians in learning from their experiences and progressing in their expertise as well as helps to ensure good service to the client. In group therapy, supervision helps group leaders to understand their groups' participants, adopt a group-oriented perspective, monitor and regulate emotion within their groups, deal with the range of feelings induced in them by their groups, and become more familiar with the relevant treatment principles and techniques (Rosenthal, 2005). Lansen and Haans (2004) identify three categories of issues most frequently addressed in the clinical supervision of trauma therapists, namely, case conceptualization, the emotional impact of the work on the therapists, and miscellaneous problems related to the management of specific situations. Regular supervision or consultation has been identified as a key element in preventing secondary or vicarious traumatization among therapists (McCann & Pearlman, 1990; Salston & Figley, 2003). Therapeutic work with trauma survivors often poses unique challenges in regard to the therapist's countertransference (see Chu, 1988, for a review). Supervision provides therapists with an opportunity to understand these reactions so that they are not enacted to the detriment of the client or the therapist. Walker (2004) points out that when two therapists co-lead a group of abuse survivors the possibility of multiple projections, transferences, and countertransferences is dramatically increased. If these issues are not recognized and addressed in supervision, they can become unmanageable and potentially destructive to the group.

The role of the supervisor for TRG is both demanding and multifaceted. The supervisor should support group leaders in implementing the key features of the treatment model in a manner that fits with their respective therapeutic styles. Perhaps most important, he or she should help the co-leaders maintain the goal focus and trauma frame that define the model and enable members to do the work of the group. Part of the supervisor's role is to keep the "big picture" in view, reminding group leaders of where they are in the overall trajectory of the group and of the work that should be taking place in each phase. The supervisor helps co-leaders attend to the progress of each member in relation to her chosen goal as well as group process issues that may enhance or hinder therapeutic work or need to be otherwise addressed. Supervision provides a forum for "troubleshooting"—addressing specific problems that may arise over the course of the group sessions (e.g., difficulty in containing a particular member, out-of-group contacts between two group members). The supervisor also plays a key role in attending to dynamics that may arise between co-leaders based on differences in power, leadership styles, or other factors. The supervisor should be actively checking in with co-leaders about these issues for the entirety of the therapy. As has already been mentioned, supervision also has an important function in reducing secondary traumatization by enabling group leaders to be "debriefed" about what members have shared and their personal reactions in a safe and confidential setting. This function is especially critical for this type of group, owing to the intensity fostered by the time limit, the typically high level of affective and interpersonal engagement that occurs within the group, and the focus on members sharing their trauma narrative in the service of a goal. The importance of having a supervisory relationship in which these issues can be processed cannot be overemphasized, regardless of the co-leaders' level of experience. It is the supervisor's responsibility to create an environment in which co-leaders feel safe to discuss their respective clinical difficulties and personal reactions as well as any conflict that arises in the dyad over the course of the sessions. Supervision is regarded as sufficiently important that it is the sole subject of a separate chapter (Chapter 7) of this treatment guide.

CRITERIA FOR GROUP MEMBERS

Although this manual describes a women-only trauma recovery group, it can easily be adapted for both co-ed and men's trauma recovery groups. Members of this group should have achieved some stability and control over trauma-related symptoms. They should have no suicidal or self-harming behavior, hospitalizations, or substance abuse for at least the preceding year. They should have some healthy coping behaviors and at least a few established social connections. They should have done some prior trauma work and ideally should be engaged in stable concurrent individual therapy (or, at the very least, have access to a previous therapist to whom they can return if needed during the group). Their current living situation should be safe, and they should not be anticipating any major life changes or crises over the course of the therapy. Furthermore, potential members should have an interest in group therapy, be able to commit to regular and punctual attendance, and be able also to articulate at least a vague goal for the group. These criteria are described in detail in the Chapter 3, on "Initial Preparations and Member Screening."

It is important that group leaders pay attention to the *overall composition* of the group. While the TRG initially began as a group for incest survivors, we have that these groups were able to tolerate a fair amount of heterogeneity in terms of trauma history (e.g., one group might include survivors whose primary traumas involve childhood sexual abuse, intimate partner violence, and adult sexual assault). Similarly, diversity among members in regard to race, ethnicity, religious background, age, and sexual orientation tends to enrich the group and underline the commonalities experienced among survivors despite their apparent differences. It is often helpful if each member has at least one other person with whom he or she can identify relatively easily, although this is not always possible. As will be discussed further in the next chapter, it is very important that a member know if she will be the only representative of a particular social group (e.g., person of color, lesbian, person with a disability) so that she can make an informed choice about her own participation.

GROUP FRAMEWORK

Group Size

Based on our experience, five to eight group members seems to be the ideal size for the typical TRG in order for participants to have the appropriate amount of sharing and feedback time to accomplish their goals. With more than eight members, it becomes very difficult to devote sufficient time to each member's therapeutic work. When there are fewer than five members, the unique benefits of a group intervention are reduced, particularly if a member is absent or drops out of treatment.

Group Length

This manual is based on a typical TRG that meets once a week for 90 minutes for 16 weeks. The length and frequency of meetings is well suited to the emotional intensity of the work. Although the duration of the therapy is flexible (ranging in our experience anywhere from 10 weeks to 8 months), it is vital to choose a specific duration and subsequently comply with that time frame. Also, it is important to be aware of the advantages and disadvantages to different therapy durations. A shorter time frame provides more focus and impetus to members' actively pursuing their goals; however, it may limit the depth of this work and often does not allow much room for processing in-group interpersonal experiences that may be relevant to members' identified goals. A longer time frame may enable members to accomplish more extended goals that may involve processing both out-of-group and in-group experiences; however, there is also the risk that members may stray unduly from their goals or procrastinate in regard to pursuing them. In order prevent this situation, staged goals (i.e., goals that are deliberately "broken down" into several increments) can be helpful in providing members with multiple motivating experiences of success. If at all possible, the group should be scheduled so as to avoid frequent or prolonged disruptions attributable to holidays or therapist vacations. Co-leaders should also be aware that holidays (e.g., Mother's Day, Thanksgiving, Valentine's Day) will inevitably introduce particular dynamics and content into the group that will need to be addressed in relation to members' treatment goals.

Group Guidelines

In order for members to work productively toward their goals, it is crucial that the group environment be experienced as a safe and containing setting. It is important for group leaders to understand (and be able to help members understand) the sometimes hazy distinction between feeling unsafe in the group and feeling challenged by the therapeutic work. Behaviors that may be experienced as abusive or as causing other members to feel unsafe to participate in the group should not be tolerated, and it is the leaders' responsibility to ensure that these boundaries are maintained and intervene promptly if they are violated. However, there are times when a client may reexperience feelings of anxiety and fear or other intense affects from the past and attribute them to the group's feeling unsafe in the present. In this instance, the leaders' role is to help the member name and explore her feelings in an effort to differentiate between past and present.

It is essential to establish and uphold a clear set of guidelines for participation in order to provide a sense of safety for group members. Some guidelines that we have found to be central to maintaining a safe and productive setting for members' therapeutic work include confidentiality, mutual respect, no out-of-group contacts with other members, no touching, no food, and advance warning about any anticipated lateness or absences. These guidelines are discussed in detail in Chapter 4.

INDIVIDUAL SESSION FORMAT

Check-In

At the start of each session, there is an opening round or group check-in that should last approximately 5–7 minutes. During check-in, clients are asked to state as briefly as possible how they are doing or feeling as they start the group. This check-in is important because it gives each group member an opportunity to have her voice heard in the room, and this in turn often inclines members to talk more freely throughout the session. During the check-in, members may also claim time to share their goal-related work.

Sharing and Feedback

The majority of the session time is divided among clients sharing and receiving feedback from other group members. In a 90-minute group with an opening and closing "round," typically three group members will be able to "claim time," with approximately 25 minutes devoted to each person for sharing her goal work and receiving feedback. It is the responsibility of group leaders to structure the sharing and feedback within each session so that each contributor has roughly an equal amount of time (unless a group member specifically states that she needs less time). Approximately halfway through each member's allotted sharing time, co-leaders should check in with her about whether it would be all right to pause in her narrative to receive feedback from other group members.

Sharing

During their allotted time for sharing, group members may talk about the painful details of their trauma histories. For some, speaking about these experiences may in itself be the focus of their therapeutic work in the group; for others, it may be a necessary part of identifying, defining, and/or contextualizing an appropriate out-of-group goal. The commonalities that emerge in regard to survivors' experiences of trauma and its impact create strong affective connections among group members and decrease feelings of isolation and shame. It is important to note, however, that disclosure should be carefully paced and guided by an awareness of each member's needs in regard to the development and pursuit of her goal.

At the start of each session, it is helpful to ask each group member to start her time taking/sharing by stating her goal insofar as it has been formulated. This approach not only helps the group member focus her sharing on matters pertinent to her goal but also assists other members of the group in providing relevant feedback.

Since most participants lead very complex lives, it is understandable that a group member might get off track and share other pressing issues that do not necessarily relate to her goal. When this situation occurs, group leaders should gently and respectfully intervene to guide the group member back to her goal work (and encourage her to address the extraneous content in individual therapy, if appropriate). This reminder is intended to be containing and instructive to the member concerned and reassuring to other members.

Group members should be encouraged to monitor their affective reactions while sharing and be attentive to cues that may lead them to start dissociating. Whenever dissociation occurs, they should utilize their coping skills to reorient themselves to the present, with support from the co-leaders and other members as needed.

Feedback

The most important guidelines for providing efficacious feedback are that it should be goal-relevant and focused on the group member who is sharing. As group members share their past experiences, there are likely to be many points of commonality that may stimulate the fresh recall of similar memories for everyone in the group. As they listen, group members will have a natural tendency to compare mentally their own experiences with those of the person who is sharing. Although having had similar experiences may help a group member to relate to the person sharing, it is crucial that any feedback remain focused on the needs and experiences of *that* person. In this regard, it is often helpful to remind group members to focus on the empathic message that they wish to convey to the person sharing rather than getting involved in describing the details of their own experiences.

It is often helpful to remind group members that making an observation or asking a question of the person who is sharing is usually more helpful than stating an opinion or giving advice. No one in the group should give feedback as an authority; rather, everyone should share their perspectives as individuals with varying experiences that can aid one another toward healing. Since learning to give helpful feedback is frequently a difficult and anxiety-provoking task for group members, it is especially essential that group leaders continuously model appropriate feedback strategies.

Usually members claim time on a *rotating basis* so that they take a turn every other session to share their goal-related work. However, it is important to have some flexibility in this regard to accommodate needs that might arise related to the work of individual members. For example, a member who uses her time one week to prepare for a disclosure or confrontation may request some time the following week to process what occurred. Alternatively, a member who is struggling emotionally during a particular session may ask for time to share when she is not scheduled to do so or may offer her time to others and participate instead in providing feedback. However, it is important that group leaders assure that time is shared roughly equally overall, that no member goes without sharing for more than two consecutive sessions, and that members who are not claiming time are still actively engaged in the group.

Closing Round

Comparable to the check-in, in reverse, the closing round provides an opportunity for everyone to say how she is feeling as she leaves the group. The closing round provides group members with an opportunity to notify the leaders if they are feeling unsafe or worried about themselves in any way. Equally as important, the closing round allows time for members to share the positive self-care strategies that they plan to engage in following the session. Group members find this exercise useful, both to remind themselves of their own resourcefulness and to give others new ideas for their self-care. Because clients are doing such intense work during the group sessions, it is important to encourage them to pay extra attention to taking care of themselves and to acknowledge and reward their hard work.

CONTINUING GROUP WORK BETWEEN SESSIONS

Structured homework exercises are not a part of TRG. However, there are several ways in which each member's goal-related work will carry over into their treatment and life outside of the group.

Out-of-Group Goals

It is often the case that group members need to complete some of their goal work outside of the group sessions. Many group members will have out-of-group goals (e.g., disclosing their abuse to a family member, setting limits in a significant relationship) and use their time in group sessions to prepare for this work, report back on their progress, and obtain feedback and support.

Self-Care

Establishing routines of self-care is a major focus of Stage 1 trauma groups. Among participants in Stage 2 groups these routines should already be reliably established, and the continuing focus should be on enhanced self-nurturing to ameliorate the emotional strain of trauma-focused work for the duration of the therapy. This requirement may involve taking extra steps to keep physically and emotionally healthy by eating well and exercising, engaging in stress-relieving activities such as yoga or meditation, making more extensive use of existing social supports, and planning enjoyable and relaxing activities such as watching a movie or taking a long bath.

Individual Therapy

Individual therapy should be used concurrently with the TRG to address issues that may arise for the client over the course of the therapy. The client's individual therapist can be an important ally in honing and specifying goals as well as processing goal-related material at a depth not possible within the framework of a time-limited group. It is important to ascertain whether the therapist will use the individual sessions to support the client's group work during the course of the group sessions—otherwise, the client may feel torn between the two processes. It may be necessary to initiate a discussion with the individual therapist on how best to work together. Individual therapy is a helpful venue for processing reactions that may be evoked by participating in the group. If these concerns are relevant to the client's selected goal, the individual therapist can assist the member in finding ways to bring them back to the group during her sharing time.

CONCLUSION

This chapter has reviewed key issues related to the purposes, key features, structure, and format of the TRG. The subsequent chapters consider their practical implementation as the reader is guided from preparation and screening, through the introductory phase and goal work, to goal completion and finally to the conclusion of the group treatment.

CHAPTER 3

Initial Preparations
and Member Screening

The preparatory phase of the TRG begins with the intention to offer this type of therapy group and includes a thorough screening process that ideally results in identifying five to eight clients appropriate for inclusion in the group who are committed to participate. Table 3.1 presents an overview of pregroup tasks for co-leaders to aid them in preparing to undertake a TRG therapy group.

As a starting point, we recommend that the two group co-leaders familiarize themselves with this treatment guide in its entirety. This therapy is not a group model that can be learned a week at a time. It is important to have a well-informed overview of the group structure at the outset so that the concept of the group can be described accurately and fully to potential clients. The group co-leaders should be comfortable working together and open to sharing their work with a supervisor. The supervisor should also be identified before group sessions begin, with regular supervision meetings scheduled to start during the recruitment and screening period. Since the screening process often presents complicated clinical challenges, careful screening of potential members is one of the keys to forming a successful group.

SCREENING

As a Stage 2 trauma-focused group, the TRG involves clients' exploring and processing relevant traumatic memories in the interest of working on a goal related to their present life. This work can evoke painful feelings of fear, anger, shame, sadness, and grief as members recall how they were victimized and mourn what was lost. It is not uncommon for group members to experience temporary worsening of symptoms (e.g., increased hypervigilance, more intrusive memories) while engaged in this work. For this reason, it is very important

TABLE 3.1. Overview of Pregroup Tasks for Co-leaders

Step 1: Personal Preparation

Before undertaking to lead a TRG, you should:

1. Familiarize yourself with this treatment guide.
2. Determine whether this model is a good fit for you and the clients with whom you work.
3. Confirm your interest in deepening your foundation of information about the impact of complex trauma on survivors and learning more about the tasks of the second stage of recovery.
4. Consider whether you are open to working in a flexible way that remains structured yet encourages goal-directed process within that framework.
5. Be committed to spending an indeterminate amount of time screening candidates for the group, followed by at least 16 weeks of group sessions.
6. Be able to identify both a co-leader and a supervisor who meet the requisite criteria.
7. Be willing to undertake immediate and ongoing efforts to work effectively and openly with your co-leader and your supervisor/consultant.
8. Establish a group meeting schedule with time, location, and tentative starting date as well as the same for supervisory meetings.

Step 2: Recruitment

1. Distribute group flyers to potential clients (see the sample provided in Appendix A) or clinicians who might provide referrals (Appendix B).
2. Contact specific agencies and colleagues to inform them about the group and thereby to generate referrals.
3. Keep an ongoing list of responses accessible to both co-leaders for follow-up.

Step 3: Screening/group formation

1. Respond by phone to clients and clinicians calling about the group. Use this call as an opportunity to prescreen the client or arrange a time to do so (see Appendix C for a sample script). Educate clinicians about appropriate referrals for this group.
2. If indicated based on the telephone prescreening, schedule an intake appointment. These are ideally done with both co-leaders present.
3. Consult with the client's therapist (see Appendix E), the group co-leader, and the supervisor, and consider the evolving group's composition before sharing the disposition of clients' inclusion requests with them.
4. Finalize the group's starting and ending dates.
5. Communicate the disposition of requests to all individuals who were screened, and confirm their availability and commitment for the entire duration of the group.

that potential members be assessed as having already established safety and stability both within themselves and in their lives, and also have good coping skills and access to appropriate supports. This baseline of safety, stability, and adequate support increases the likelihood that the client will experience success and a sense of mastery in the group therapy. If this key baseline is lacking, a member's participation may lead her to feel more overwhelmed, disempowered, and isolated. Including a group member who is not ready for Stage 2 work can also threaten the security of the group as a whole, as other clients may worry about the member's ability to manage her distress or her potentially engaging in unsafe behavior. Consequently, we strongly recommend that group leaders invest sufficient time and energy in screening potential group members, and that they resist the temptation to include clients who do not meet the criteria described in this chapter.

During the screening process, group leaders should combine information obtained from the client, the referring clinician, medical records, and other sources to assess whether a good match exists between the goals and structure of the group and the client's current treatment strengths and needs. This process involves gathering relevant background data so that group leaders can assess the client's "fit" with the group structure and evolving cohort as well as educating the client and her individual therapist about the group so that they can make an informed decision about whether she should participate. We have found that it is best to frame the screening as a type of consultation. If at the end of the consultation group leaders determine that this group is not an appropriate treatment option for the client, they can use the opportunity to make recommendations about more suitable groups or other steps that could be taken to further foster her recovery.

Our usual intake process involves brief initial telephone screening followed by an in-person interview if it seems as though there may be a suitable match between the client and group. Although it is not usually feasible for the co-leaders to interview every client together, we recommend that they do so whenever possible. Co-conducting the initial interview communicates to the client a collaborative and unified relationship between the co-leaders, and it affords both co-leaders an opportunity to experience the client "in the room" in a way that is hard to replicate through other means.

The group leaders then initiate collateral contacts with the referring clinician and others involved in the client's care. Once they have gathered all relevant information, conducted the interview(s), and consulted with each other and the group supervisor/consultant, the group leaders jointly decide group membership and then communicate their decision to each potential client and referring clinician. We discuss each of these components of the screening process in detail below.

Telephone Prescreening

We recommend that the group leader first conduct a telephone prescreening with each potential client to assess whether she meets the basic criteria for a group of this nature. This preliminary contact can conserve time and save on costs involved in bringing someone in for an in-person interview when there is clearly a poor match. It may also reveal specific areas that need to be elucidated further in an in-person interview or collateral contacts.

The phone screening should begin with communicating to the client that the purpose of the phone interview is both to give her some basic information about the TRG and to find out more about what she is looking for in group treatment. The phone screening is thus an opportunity for the group leader to provide introductory psychoeducation about the group and determine whether the client meets the most basic criteria for participation in a group of this kind. We review the specific criteria in greater detail in the next section, but they include the following:

1. The client is currently not living in an unsafe situation.
2. Her symptoms are relatively stable and manageable.
3. She has done some prior trauma work and has access to an individual therapist.
4. She has not engaged in suicidal or actively self-harming behavior within the past year.
5. She has not abused substances within the past year.
6. She is not anticipating any major life changes over the course of the group sessions.
7. She is able to commit to reliable attendance.

After the initial phone screening, if the group leaders determine that the client clearly does not seem appropriate for this group and has failed to meet one or more of the basic criteria, she should be referred to a different group if a better match is available. In Appendix C, we include a complete sample script, data-collecting outline, and checklist (including an outcome-tracking component) for the telephone prescreening interview.

Intake Interview

Introduction to the Consultation

The purpose of the screening interview is to provide the potential client with comprehensive information about the group and to find out more about her life circumstances and her interest in group treatment. The objectives are to determine whether the TRG would be a good match for the client at this time and, if so, to begin to identify possible treatment goals. We usually give the client the option to start the interview either by sharing some information about herself or by having the co-leaders describe the group. Even in these small details, from the very outset group leaders offer prospective clients choices that lessen the power imbalance and give them opportunities to shape the course of the consultation.

Description of the Group

If the client asks first for more information about the group or who may be in it, leaders might respond as follows:

> "This is a group for women survivors who have suffered from the effects of violence and abuse, either in childhood or more recently. We consider violence against women to be a violation of basic human rights. With the support of the group and the co-leaders, each member chooses and works on a goal that is related to her trauma and relevant to her present life. Defining and accomplishing this goal is an important way to regain a sense of power and self-respect; having this experience in a group is an important way to regain a sense of community. In preparing for or doing their goal work, members usually share their trauma histories in some detail.
>
> "There are usually about six members in the group and two co-leaders. The group will meet once a week on [day and time period] for 90 minutes for a period of 4 months.

Group sessions begin with a brief check-in by all members and end with a closing round. The remainder of the time is shared by usually three members who describe working on their goals and receive feedback from the others, with alternating turns each week. Members of the group typically have experienced a variety of traumas. All potential members participate in the same intake process, and careful consideration is given to bringing together a group of survivors who are ready and able to do trauma-focused work. This group is for women who have done some trauma work in previous therapy. While members may still struggle with symptoms, they should feel relatively safe and stable in their lives. Members should not have recently engaged in any high-risk behavior or be expecting any major life changes during the treatment period, as active participation in the group can stir up painful feelings that may require con-siderable emotional energy. Members should have some established coping skills that they can employ if symptoms become stressful. Members should be able to imagine talking about their trauma and listening to others describe theirs without becoming overwhelmed. We'd be happy to share more specific details with you after we answer your questions."

If the client prefers to begin the intake consultation by being interviewed, the infor-mation above should be conveyed immediately afterward or interspersed throughout the interview. Introducing TRG therapy in this way provides prospective clients with a basic understanding of the screening process and makes them aware that co-leaders are carefully considering the safety and stability of the group as a whole as well as that of individual members in making decisions about inclusion.

Gathering Background Information

The group leaders should spend the remainder of the session gathering information from the client to determine whether the group is a good match with her treatment needs and strengths. While there is no set format for conducting the interview, the general areas that they should assess include the reason for referral to the group, current life circumstances, psychiatric history (including current treatment), and trauma history. Over the course of the interview (and through collateral contacts with other treatment professionals), group leaders should obtain specific information about the criteria described in detail below and outlined in Appendix D, the screening interview checklist.

CURRENT INTEREST IN GROUP THERAPY

It is important in inquire about the potential client's current interest in group therapy. For starters, one must ensure that the client's interests and expectations for group therapy are congruent with the TRG treatment model. Sometimes a client has little personal interest in group therapy and is being compliant because her therapist referred her to the group. Although it is important for the client's individual therapist to support group therapy, it is *vital* that the client have a vested personal interest in the group as well. Occasionally, clients want to "have their story heard" because they believe it will benefit other survivors. It is far more important that potential group members come to the group because they hope that it will make a difference in their own lives.

INDIVIDUAL THERAPY

Because the violation of basic human rights damages the capacity for trusting relationships, safety and self-care depend on the establishment of a reliable relational matrix. The TRG is part of this matrix, but it is not a standalone treatment model. To provide adequate support for the emotionally intense work of this group, preferably the client should also be involved in an ongoing, stable, and productive individual therapy, in which she has already done some significant exploratory work on her trauma history. The goals of her individual therapy should be both consistent and in synch with the goals of the group, and group leaders should be able to have a constructive collaborative relationship with the individual therapist.

A conflict may occasionally arise when a client whose individual therapy is focused primarily on symptom management expresses an interest in participating in a trauma processing group (such as ours) that may temporarily worsen some of her symptoms. Problems may also arise when a therapist makes a referral to the group in order to avoid dealing with the trauma in individual therapy or in order to obtain help with a therapy that has developed boundary problems or reached an impasse. To gain a better understanding of the status of the client's individual therapy, one must obtain information from both the client and therapist. Sample questions for the client may include the following:

"What is the focus of the work you that you are currently doing in individual therapy?"
"Have you spoken to your current therapist about participating in this group?"

It is essential that the client understand that there will be communications between the group leaders and the individual therapist over the entire course of the TRG treatment.

In the rare instance in which a client is not in current individual therapy but has been in the past and meets all of the other criteria, she may still participate in the group if she has access to a previous therapist and is able and willing to re-engage in therapy if needed. Occasionally, other strong relational supports such as a well-established recovery fellowship may serve the same function.

PREVIOUS TRAUMA-FOCUSED WORK

The client should have previously done some trauma-focused work in individual and/or group therapy. Clients should have experienced sharing the details of their trauma with at least one other person and should be able to anticipate sharing with the group and listening to others do the same. Group leaders should probe for specific ways in which the client's trauma history has been addressed in her therapy. Having the client provide some basic details about her trauma history is an important component of the intake interview, not only to gather necessary information but also to assess how the client manages the experience of sharing it with the group leaders. If a client avoids talking about her trauma history during the interview or becomes highly activated when doing so, this group would clearly not be an appropriate treatment choice. In one screening interview, for example, a client was unable to answer any questions about her trauma history without becoming tearful and distraught. She revealed that she had not talked about her trauma history in any detail with her therapist. The group leaders recommended that she attempt this in her individual therapy as preparation for a future group. Sample questions about prior trauma work include the following:

> "Have you done any work on your trauma in past treatments?"
> "How has the experience of working on your trauma in therapy been for you?"
> "To what extent have you spoken about your trauma history with your current therapist?"
> "What kinds of issues have you been working on in therapy in relation to your trauma?"

Asking clients to provide some basic details about their trauma histories also provides the group leaders with information that is important in understanding the overall group composition and its potential dynamics, to prevent a situation in which one member feels isolated or alienated from the group. For example, a member who was sexually abused by a sibling close in age may experience confusion about the validity of her abuse relative to other members whose abusers were adult caretakers. Similarly, a client with a particularly extreme history (e.g., involving experiences such as imprisonment, torture, forced prostitution, or severe injuries) may feel alone and different in a group of survivors with "milder" and more common forms of interpersonal trauma. We have also found that sexually abused women with female perpetrators worry about being "the only one" and judged by other group members for being different. This potential for alienation can be addressed by trying to ensure that there is at least one other person who has something in common with this member. Ideally, the other person should share some aspect of her history, since past trauma is particularly salient in a Stage 2 group; but, if this is not possible, commonality on some other important dimension (e.g., ethnic background, sexual orientation, occupation) may serve a similar purpose.

It is important that group leaders encourage clients to give prior thought to how they may be affected both by sharing their stories with others and hearing about others' trauma histories. Important questions to ask in every screening interview thus include:

> "What do you think it would be like to talk about your trauma with a group of other women?"
> "What do you think it would be like to hear about the traumatic events that other members have experienced?"

When asked the latter question, one woman in a screening interview reflected on how her yoga training had helped her learn to protect her mood, and so she would not get overwhelmed by others' experience. At an earlier point in time, this woman might have become quite overwhelmed by hearing other women's trauma histories, but she had since developed some healthy coping strategies upon which she could draw. Thus, regarding this criterion, this woman seemed like a good prospective fit for the TRG.

COPING SKILLS

The client should have in place some healthy coping techniques that she can rely on when she feels emotionally distressed. These skills are vital to modulate the intense affect that can be evoked during this type of group, and potential members should be educated about their importance. In the initial interview, it is important to ask questions to determine whether the client has sufficient coping skills to manage the intensity of a Stage 2 recovery group without resorting to self-harming behaviors. Sample questions include:

> "What are some of the things that you have in your life that you use to take care of yourself or cope with stress?"
> "When you are having a bad day, what is the worst that things get for you? How do you get through it?"

In our screening interviews, women often mention meditation, painting, poetry, breathing exercises, reaching out to friends and family, exercise, and working as some examples of ways in which they cope with difficult feelings. The following dialogue illustrates the creative ways in which one client expressed coping with day-to-day stressors:

THERAPIST: What do you do to cope on your worst day?

CLIENT: There are still hard days, but now I have better coping skills; so, I don't let it upset me for the whole day. And I do the meditation thing. There are a lot of things that I do. And maybe there is a painting that I do, and when I do it I am taken away completely.

THERAPIST: It sounds like your coping skills really help—the meditation and the painting.

CLIENT: Yes. I used to do poetry only when I was sad. Now I write whether I am happy or I am sad. I am not going to say that the depression does not come back. It does; it's just that it is like a friend or an enemy who comes to visit me, and I have to decide how to interact with it. That's something I have to accept. I have moved on.

THERAPIST: It sounds like you have really made a lot of progress.

CLIENT: Therapy has really helped me.

SOCIAL SUPPORTS

Although clients in this group often struggle with feeling isolated, they should have at least some social network or people in their lives other than their individual therapist to whom they can turn when in need of support (e.g., family, friends, religious community, recovery fellowship). The presence of at least a few social connections also suggests that the client has some basic interpersonal skills that are important for participating in a group. Questions to ask about social supports include the following:

> "Through the groups you have joined or through other means, have you been able to establish any kinds of support in your life?"
> "Do you have any friends or other people with whom you maintain contact and can turn to for support?"
> "Have you spoken with any of them about your trauma history? If so, how did they react?"

In general, it is important for the therapist to inquire about supports in some detail if the client is vague about them. If it becomes clear that the client has no one other than her therapist that she can identify as a source of support, and she is looking to the group to be a primary source of support, other types of groups (e.g., ongoing support groups or social groups) are likely to be more appropriate. A client lacking outside supports is likely to become frustrated and overwhelmed in the TRG, and other members may be forced to react by taking on unneeded burdens of care taking and concern, distracting them unduly from their own goal work.

NO RECENT PSYCHIATRIC HOSPITALIZATIONS

As an indication of their stability, clients should not have required inpatient psychiatric care during the preceding year. If the client has participated in a partial hospital or day treatment program, elicit the reasons for and nature of the admission to determine whether this involvement would preclude participation in the group.

NO RECENT SUICIDAL OR SELF-HARMING BEHAVIOR

Clients may still experience suicidal ideation and/or self-harming urges, but they should not have acted on such thoughts and impulses within the past year, and they should have several alternative techniques for managing distressing affect. Bingeing and purging or denial associated with an eating disorder may also constitute self-harming behavior, and the risk of potential exacerbation during a trauma-focused group needs to be examined with the client and her therapist. Sample questions include the following:

> "Within the past year, how often have you struggled with thoughts about wanting to hurt or kill yourself?"
> "Have there been times when you have acted on these thoughts?"

"What has prevented you from acting on those thoughts and urges?"
"What do you do instead to manage your feelings?"

One client responded:

"I've struggled with suicidal thoughts for many years. I think they made me feel like I had an out if I needed it, you know? But I've worked with my therapist a lot on not having that be an option for me anymore. Taking it off the table. So, I haven't been in the hospital for over 4 years. I have fleeting thoughts sometimes when I'm very stressed, but I know I would never act on them."

Thus, it appears that the client has actively worked on her chronic thoughts of suicide with her therapist and has in fact stayed safe for a significant amount of time. Based on this criterion, therefore, she would be a good prospective group member. Follow-up questions might address her positive reasons for staying alive and the security of her social support system. When in doubt, we recommend not including potentially suicidal patients in the group.

NO RECENT SUBSTANCE ABUSE

The client should not have engaged in substance abuse for at least the past year. In assessing substance use, it is important to consider not only quantity and frequency but also the client's motivation for using and its impact. For clients with a history of substance abuse or dependence, it is important to evaluate how much support they have in regard to maintaining their sobriety as well as the presence of alternative coping skills. Sample questions include:

"Have you or anyone else been concerned about your substance use during the past year?"
"Are there still times when you feel urges to use?"
"What helps you through at those times?"

A client appropriate for inclusion in this group might respond:

"I think I'll always feel urges to use at certain points. But what helps me is remembering what else comes with that—all the chaos. I can't even imagine having my life be like that again—I have too much to lose now. My home, my kids. So, if I feel tempted to use, I call my sponsor and talk to her. I attend more meetings that week."

This type of response indicates that the client recognizes that the urge to use substances will be a continuing vulnerability for her and that she has given thought to the risks of using substances and has a clear plan to obtain support if she needs to do so. In general, inquiring about a client's history of relapse, if any, helps establish what circumstances promote vulnerability. For example, if a client reports having relapsed when she worked on difficult material in therapy, the TRG may not be the best fit for her at this juncture.

NO ACTIVE OR RECENT PSYCHOSIS

The client may have experienced psychotic symptoms at some point in her history but currently does not have a primary psychotic disorder. The client should have a history of treatment compliance, and symptoms should be responsive to medication.

SAFE ENVIRONMENT

The client's current living circumstances should be physically and emotionally safe (e.g., not caring for a perpetrating parent; not at imminent risk of losing her housing). Clients' current relationships should not be violent, abusive, or retraumatizing in any way. Example of questions co-leaders can ask include:

> "Do you currently have any concerns about your safety?"
> "What is the quality of your current relationship?"
> "Do you worry about being physically or emotionally harmed by your partner?"
> "Has your partner been supportive of your healing process?"
> "Do you currently have any contact with the person(s) who abused you? If so, what is the nature of that contact?"

In one screening interview, a client who discussed being in a time of transition in her life referred to a relationship that was (until very recently) emotionally and physically abusive, which she appeared to be tolerating to some extent. The therapist inquired about the last incident of abuse, about help the client's partner was getting, and about the client's current understanding of the relationship. The goal in general is not just to explore the safety of the relationship but also, if there have been concerns, the extent to which the client is aware of their implications and what steps have been taken to address them. The therapist inquired about the safety of the client's child and what legal issues were at play. Eventually, this client was not screened into the group because it was clear that the abuse was recent, and, since her partner was ambivalent about getting help, she thus continued to worry for her safety. In another interview, when the therapist inquired about the custody arrangements of a client's children, the client revealed that her ex-husband was controlling and difficult. The therapist then explored the issue of physical violence in the relationship and how much contact the client had with her ex-husband. It became clear that she did not appear to be at risk for current violence and had taken steps to increase her emotional safety. She was thus screened into the group.

NO PENDING MAJOR LIFE CHANGES

The client should not be anticipating major changes and stressors over the course of the group therapy (e.g., testifying in court, major surgery). Such life events require that the individual have full access to her emotional resources and intact coping skills, which could be temporarily compromised by the intensity of the uncovering work that occurs in this kind of group. Such life events might also compromise her attendance at group sessions, which would have an impact on the group as a whole. The co-leaders might ask: "Are you anticipating any major life changes in the next 6 months?" More moderate life changes (e.g., moving one's residence, a son or daughter leaving for college) do not necessarily preclude inclusion in this group, but it is it is important to consider whether the client has a strong enough support system and established coping skills to assist her through this transition while participating in the group. In some instances a life change (e.g., a child leaving home) may become incorporated into her goal.

CLIENT IS ABLE TO ARTICULATE A POSSIBLE GOAL

Clients should be able to understand the concept of a goal and the rationale for making the goal a central focus of the group therapy. The purpose of the individual goal is both to provide a structure and focus for the client's group participation and to promote a sense of mastery and self-efficacy. The screening interview is an opportunity to introduce the idea of a goal to prospective group members, as well as some guidelines for identifying one that is suitable for the group, so that the client can think about it further and discuss it with her individual therapist. The client need not commit to a goal at this preliminary stage; rather, group leaders should look for a predisposition to consider possible goals and to understand how particular goals in the present might be related to traumatic experiences in the past. As we discussed in detail in Chapter 2, we encourage clients to choose a goal related to their trauma history and affecting their current lives. In addition, clients are told that goals should be specific rather than broad, concrete and measurable rather than abstract, and realistically achievable within the time limits of the therapy. The following are sample questions for assessing these dimensions of a potential goal:

> How do you understand the connection of this problem with your history of trauma?" (trauma-related)
> "In what ways is your life still affected by your trauma? What would be something you would want to change in that area?" (present-oriented)
> "How would you know if you accomplished that goal? How would your daily life look different?" (concrete)
> "Is there a particular area of your life in which you are experiencing this problem most acutely? How is it affecting you in this area?" (specific)
> "That sounds like an important but very large goal. What piece of it might be achievable within the time frame of the group?" (realistic)

The group leaders explain the collaborative nature of goal setting and the ways in which goals may be honed or expanded over the course of the therapy. Some examples of in- and out-of-group goals may be provided. The following examples illustrate how the co-leaders address goal formation in the screening interview:

THERAPIST: Maybe we could talk a little bit about goals. An important aspect of this group is coming up with a goal that one can work on during the group. The reason we have a goal-oriented format is that we want people to leave the group feeling as if they have achieved or mastered something. The goal should be something that could realistically happen in that time frame. We ask group members to choose something related to their trauma history that they are struggling with in their present lives. And we encourage people to choose something pretty specific. Do you have a sense of what a goal for you might be in the group?

CLIENT: I want to have a healthy relationship with a man. I come into relationships feeling as if they are all powerful and they are up there and I am down here.

THERAPIST: It sounds like a really good starting place, and many women come into this group with a similar goal. The next step would be to make it more specific and narrow it down to something you could begin working on. In a 4-month group, you may not be able to accomplish the whole goal, but there may be an important step toward that goal that you could work on during the course of the sessions. For example, you might want to start by trying to identify some things that come up when you get into a relationship with a man.

CLIENT: I think I am afraid that I will not be accepted just the way I am.

THERAPIST: Right, so that could be a good place to begin. You could talk about it further with your individual therapist, and it is something the group could also be helpful in figuring out—how to translate an insight like that into a goal that you could accomplish.

In this example, the therapist begins by describing the purposes and characteristics of a group goal and eliciting the client's thoughts about what she is hoping to achieve. The client starts out with a goal that does not seem realistic for a 4-month group. The group leader provides further psychoeducation about the process of breaking a large goal into incremental steps and encourages her to begin thinking about some of the issues that arise at the beginning of a new relationship. After identifying some of these concerns, the next step would be to help her find a way to operationalize them into a concrete goal. This approach may be part of the group process for this client, during which the group leaders and other group members may aid her in setting an achievable goal for the group. Another example of narrowing down a group goal follows:

THERAPIST: You asked if a person could do two goals, and we usually stick with one— although we sometimes do serial goals, so things get broken down into steps.

CLIENT: When I think about all the things that I want to do, they all have to do with the one goal of becoming less isolated.

THERAPIST: So, it sounds like maybe trying to find a way to make that as concrete as possible in regard to what piece of it you could work on in a 4-month group is our best approach. We try to help people to have a goal that feels concrete so that you can know if you have achieved it or not. So, for example, it might involve reaching out to one or more people or involving yourself in particular activities that would put you into contact with more people. As you think about it, you may find that you come up with other ideas. This initial consultation is usually a place where things just start to percolate, and people often find that their ideas become clearer as time goes on. Once the group starts, other group members may also be able to help you come up with some concrete ideas about how to become less isolated.

In this example, the client had several different goals she wanted to work on, and the therapist helped her to start contemplating ways in which these goals may be related to one another. The group leader also urged the client to think about ways of making her goal of being less isolated more concrete so that she would know if and when she accomplished it. She provided some examples of this process but also left open the possibility that the client would come with her own ideas, perhaps with some feedback from the group.

In thinking about the group's overall composition, it is important that the majority of group members be able to identify one or two reasonably clear areas of focus for their goal, even though the specific goal might only be finalized during the early sessions of the group. It is possible to include one or two members who are less certain of the specific goals during the screening process; but having more than that can derail the group if members take an excessively long time to decide upon their goals, experiencing frustration and shame when it becomes clear that they cannot achieve the goals in the remaining time.

COMMITMENT TO RELIABLE ATTENDANCE

Given the time-limited nature of the therapy and the importance of creating a safe and predictable environment for the therapeutic work, it is essential that members attend sessions regularly and punctually. Group leaders should explain these expectations, and their rationale during the initial intake interview, and clients should be asked whether they are able to make this commitment of their time and energy. Again, it is best to frame this commitment as an assertion of power and control that each client makes both on her own behalf and as a gift to the other participants. Clients too often enter the group with little understanding of how critically important their participation is to other group members.

During the screening interview, a member will occasionally notify group leaders that she will have to miss a particular session if included in the group owing to a preexisting commitment. We strongly recommend that members not miss the first two sessions or last two sessions, as we have found that missing these sessions is both a major loss for the individual member and is unnecessarily disruptive and potentially upsetting for others in the group.

Concluding the Intake Interview

At the conclusion of the interview, it is important to check in with the client to see how she is feeling after talking about the trauma she experienced in the past and to appreciate the courage it has taken to do so. She should be reminded that her intake experience might evoke even more feelings after it concludes. She should be asked to identify a self-care strategy that she could utilize to self-soothe, should the need occur. The client should be given the opportunity to ask any questions she has or to mention anything that she feels is important that was not covered in the interview. Group leaders should also obtain the required releases of information to communicate with the client's individual therapist and others involved in her treatment who may be able to provide information relevant to the referral.

With some clients, it may be immediately apparent that this group is not best suited to their needs at the intake time. The co-leaders should use this opportunity to share this information with the client in a manner that does not shame her, explaining the thought process behind this decision. If possible, alternative groups or individual treatment options can be recommended. For example, in a screening interview it was evident that the client was still highly symptomatic and had just recently begun seeing a new therapist. The co-leaders communicated to her that she might benefit more from a symptom management group at this point, and they then recommended an appropriate referral. Another client revealed that she would be starting cancer treatment during the group and was unsure about whether she would feel well enough to attend all the sessions. On the basis of both her pending health-related stress and inability to commit to regular attendance, the client was encouraged to participate in a cancer support group and encouraged to contact the group leaders to discuss inclusion in a later group once her medical condition had stabilized and she was in a better position to engage in trauma-focused work.

Collateral Contacts

Contact with the referring clinician and other providers as needed is a very important part of the screening process to gather collateral information and determine how well the group will fit in with the client's other treatments. When the client attends the screening interview, group leaders should ask her to sign a release of information to enable reciprocal communication between them and her individual therapist and/or other clinicians for the duration of the group therapy. Appendix E identifies the specific subject matter that should be covered in contacts with these professionals. The client's therapist should be asked about the history of his or her therapy, its focus, the strength of their therapeutic alliance, and the client's typical use of the therapist in crises situations. The group leader should fully explain the nature of TRG therapy and elicit the therapist's opinion about whether such a group treatment would be helpful to his or her client at this time. This exchange is also an opportunity to assess whether the individual and group therapists have a shared understanding of trauma work as it pertains to this client as well as compatible treatment goals. If this is the case and her therapist supports the client's participation in the group, the group leader should explain the purpose of the goal and the guidelines for formulating it and request that the therapist work with the client to help make it more concrete and specific.

Although collateral contact with the client's individual therapist is usually an invaluable source of information, it is important to bear in mind that clients can present quite differently in group settings than they do one-on-one. If the client has been involved in other group treatments, it can be extremely helpful to speak with the co-leader of the previous group about his or her experience of the client's participation. An issue that sometimes arises is the client's simultaneous involvement in several groups as well as individual therapy. In such a case, it is important to assess whether joining a new group would add anything different to the client's treatment or whether it may be more helpful for the client to work on expanding her social network and sphere of activities *outside* of a therapeutic context.

It is important to explain to the client that permission to communicate with her individual therapist will extend to the entirety of the group therapy. This arrangement assures the patient that all treatment agents are actively cooperating in her care. Typically, group leaders make contact with the client's individual therapist during the screening period, at the midpoint, and toward the end of the group therapy; however, if they have concerns about the client, they may call the therapist at any time (after first notifying the client). Similarly, if the individual therapist has concerns or questions, he or she may contact the group leaders at any point during the group therapy.

Communicating the Outcome of Consultations

Once group leaders have gathered the necessary information, they should consult with each other and their supervisor/consultant and decide whether a good match exists between the prospective client and group at this time. As we have already noted, it is also helpful to pay close attention to the group's overall composition in making membership decisions. In this regard, co-leaders should consider similarities and differences among the members and their potential impact on each individual's likely experience as well as the group dynamics. While being "the only one" in a particular category is certainly not sufficient a reason to automatically exclude someone, it is nonetheless important that every potential group member know in advance whether she is going to be the only person of a particular race/lesbian/younger woman/domestic violence survivor/victim of a female perpetrator, etc., so that she can make an informed decision about whether to participate. In such cases, we would acknowledge how this might make her feel different, at least initially, and let her know what efforts we would make to try to ensure that she felt part of the group. If she decided to opt out, we would support her decision and try to help her find a group that would be a more comfortable match. We have not yet been confronted with the complex question of how best to meet the needs of transgender survivors in the context of a single-gender group; however, as gender identity issues become more visible and subject to open dialogue, we anticipate that this issue will arise. We recommend that, in addition to conducting the thorough screening process described in this chapter, group leaders seek consultation from professionals and organizations with expertise in working with transgender clients.

Based on co-leader discussions, supervision, and/or collateral contact with the client's individual therapist, it sometimes becomes clear that more information is needed to answer specific questions in deciding whether the group is a good match for the client. In such instances, one should invite the client to return for a follow-up screening appointment. For example, in one case a client had lost custody of her children 2 years previously. The supervisor was concerned about including her in the group without knowing more about the circumstances surrounding this occurrence in the event that she had been abusive, as this possibility could be very upsetting to other members. In another case, the co-leaders held a second meeting with a potential member who was a survivor of particularly brutal ritualistic abuse to determine whether she would be able to do focused work without having the details of her history potentially overwhelm other members. In both of these cases, the group leaders considered the ways in which a particular member's experiences might well impact others in the group.

Group leaders should communicate the outcome of their consultations to the client promptly and directly, either in person or by telephone. For the client for whom the group is deemed inappropriate, the group leader should begin by acknowledging appreciation for her interest in the group and the work that she had done to lead her to consider this type of group. Then the leader should communicate the reasoning for the decision and provide the client with an opportunity to ask questions and express her feelings about the decision. If it is apparent that the poor match is mainly attributable to poor timing (e.g., the client has just begun individual therapy, is in the midst of a divorce, or had a relapse during the past 6 months), the group leader should encourage her to re-interview for the group in the future. The group leader should take time to inform the client about other more appropriate group offerings if these are available and make referral suggestions whenever possible. Alternatively, the group leader should provide the client with ideas regarding other steps that might be taken to prepare her for a group of this type in the future (e.g., working on her sobriety, working with her therapist to better manage her symptoms, engaging in activities that will expand her social network). She should also communicate the outcome of the consultation and any recommendations to the referring clinician.

For the client who is offered a place in the group, the leader should remind her of such details as the starting date and venue of the group, if these are known. Since launching a psychotherapy group often takes longer than anticipated, maintaining regular contact with group members prior to the start and keeping them updated of any changes are important to do. By doing so, group leaders also stay informed of whether there are any changes in members' availability or interest. Once the starting date is established, check in briefly with each member and/or referring clinician about whether there have been any changes in the client's circumstances, especially if there has been a protracted screening phase. In one case, a member had become involved in a legal case related to her trauma between the time of her screening appointment and the start of the group. The co-leaders became aware of this important development only after group sessions were under way and the member had become highly symptomatic.

Given the detailed screening process and relatively specific inclusion criteria, the preparatory phase can take quite a long time. Based on our experience, delaying the starting date of a group or conducting a smaller group is a wiser course than including a client for whom the group is a questionable or poor match. Not surprisingly, we have found that a disproportionately large number "errors" in screening occur with the last clients interviewed, when group leaders are especially anxious to get the group under way. These last-minute decisions frequently result in difficult challenges for the client, the group, and the co-leaders. In sum, the more time and attention that are invested in the screening process, the more likely the group will be a successful and rewarding experience for all concerned.

CONCLUSION

This chapter has reviewed important considerations in preparing to offer the TRG and the process of screening potential members for their individual readiness and "fit" for the group. Once group leaders have identified a group of five to eight members who meet these criteria, the group is ready to begin. The following chapters describe the implementation of TRG therapy over the three phases: the introductory sessions, goal work, and the concluding sessions.

CHAPTER 4

The Introductory Phase

The first five or six sessions of TRG therapy orient group participants to the key elements of the group by (1) providing psychoeducation about the group's purposes and structure and introducing operational guidelines; (2) beginning to establish a sense of safety and trust among the group's members; and (3) deepening the process of refining members' individual goals. The first and second sessions vary somewhat from the overall pattern in that in these two sessions the co-leaders take time to review and clarify what group members should expect in the group, undertake an "introductions exercise," and discuss guidelines for participation. Unlike subsequent sessions, these sessions have a specially prepared agenda defined by the co-leaders, who also provide much of the content. In addition to providing group members with important information about the group, this introductory process relieves initial anxiety about entering the group by enabling members to bring their voices and experiences into the room in a gradual way. Sessions 3–5 primarily involve establishing goals, and although the group leaders remain active in providing structure, focus, direction, and time management, the actual content begins to be based on the ideas that members bring into the group. The task of defining a goal may be achieved quickly by some members, but that task frequently extends beyond the fifth session for others. This chapter details the beginning phase of this process, which continues into the goal-work period of the group (discussed in Chapter 5). Although the time required to establish a clear and definable goal varies, what is most important is that it be achievable prior to the termination phase.

Before the first group session, the co-leaders should divide up the agenda for the session, determining who will take the primary organizational responsibility for each element. For example, Leader A might lead the discussion of group guidelines, while Leader B might organize and explain the introductory exercise. Of course, the emphasis on co-leadership and collaboration should be exemplified throughout, but this division of primary responsibilities helps to maintain a greater sense of organization, thereby reducing anxiety for group members. In addition, the integration of divided yet collaborative responsibility ensures that both co-leaders have active roles and helps to model the safe sharing of perceived and real power differentials from the outset of the therapy.

We present the first and second sessions here in a format closely resembling the actual group process. This approach facilitates planning and helps group leaders establish the time frame within which the TRG is implemented. We recommend following these group outlines as presented, which may require focusing on both time constraints and the format itself. Naturally, the exact wording and the style of presentation will be largely determined by the style of the co-leaders themselves. From the third session through the termination phase, sessions will follow the standard check-in, goal work, and closing round format discussed in Chapter 2. We present an overview of the session format for the introductory phase in Table 4.1. Common challenges that arise during the introductory phase of TRG are discussed toward the end of this chapter.

SESSION 1

The first session is very task-oriented, consisting chiefly of (1) welcoming and introducing members, (2) beginning to develop the group guidelines and structure, and (3) establishing a goal focus by asking members to begin to describe their goal ideas in a general way. Co-leaders typically invite members into the group room at the same time. The room contains chairs for all members and the co-leaders prearranged in a circle, easily accessible tissues,

---

TABLE 4.1. Overview of the Session Format for the Introductory Phase

Session 1

- Initial welcome and opening round
- Orientation to agenda and general group overview
- Discussion of group guidelines
- Introductions exercise
- Initial statement of goals
- Closing round

Session 2

- Opening round
- Individualized goals
- Guidelines for sharing and feedback
- Time taking
- Closing round

Sessions 3–5

- Opening round
- Time taking
- Closing round

---

and the setting has been made as comfortable as possible in terms of such factors as the lighting, temperature, and assured privacy with minimal disruptions. Co-leaders should also prepare any disability accommodations requested by individual members (e.g., a path and space for a member arriving in a wheelchair). Co-leaders typically sit across from each other to maximize the visual perspective of the members and to facilitate co-leader communication. The following is an outline of a typical first session.

Initial Welcome and Opening Round

The key components of this part of the session include the co-leaders' introducing themselves and acknowledging the group members' accomplishment in taking the big first step of coming to the group. The group leaders also provide a general overview of the first session, including the ways in which it will differ from future sessions. They then describe the opening check-in round and invite members to participate.

This first group session is unique, as it begins with the co-leaders taking time to talk before a check-in round begins. In the sample dialogue below, note the many instances of psychoeducation where group culture and expectations are described. These explanations expand upon the cognitive framework for the group provided during the screening process and occur frequently during the early stages of the therapy. This important introduction is typically split between the two co-leaders, as indicated below.

CO-LEADER 1: Welcome, everybody. I am Marjorie, and I see some familiar faces and some new faces. I sense that there are many feelings in the room and appreciate the challenge it may have taken for you to get here. Starting a group of this kind is very anxiety-producing for most people.

CO-LEADER 2: Yes, congratulations to all of you for making it here tonight—it is wonderful to see you all! I am Daphne. [Both co-leaders speak early in the process; both acknowledge the challenge and success of attending the first session.]

CO-LEADER 1: We will have a very full and different session tonight so that we can explain and begin to practice how the group will typically run and—very importantly—so that each of you can begin to get to know one another and practice talking together in preparation for goal work. Daphne and I will be talking a lot more than usual during the first few sessions. Daphne will outline how we typically begin each group, which is with a check-in or opening round.

CO-LEADER 2: The check-in is a brief opportunity—just a minute or so—for each of you to say a sentence or two about how you feel as you start each session. It is meant to help you to transition into the session, and to bring your very important voice into the room. For example, you may want to share a feeling that you are having or describe what kind of day you are experiencing. For the first several weeks we will also remind you to include your name each time you speak. It is very important that every group member participate in this opening round in whatever brief way you can. So, let's start with our brief opening round, or check-in.

CO-LEADER 1: Who would like to start?

SARA: I guess I can. My name is Sara. I am glad to be here, but a little anxious.

NANCY: My name is Nancy, and I'm feeling edgy today, not sure what to expect.

SUSANNA: My name is Susanna, and on my way here I thought, "What on earth am I doing?" And I almost turned back . . . I guess you could say I'm scared, but glad I came.

MARIA: I'm Maria. I can totally relate to how everyone is feeling. I am trying hard to stay focused.

JESS: I feel fine, just not too sure about being here tonight. Oh, I'm Jess.

LISA: I am Lisa, and I had a busy day at school—so it may take me a while to transition tonight.

In the first couple of sessions, a group leader may respond to these kinds of statements by group members by normalizing the variety of feelings mentioned and validating members' anxiety or fears about the unknown. It may also be necessary for a group leader to step in and help a member to focus and shorten their check-in. We describe this process in greater detail in the "Common Challenges" section at the end of the chapter.

Orientation to Agenda and General Group Overview

Following check-in, co-leaders provide an overview of what will be covered during this first session as well as the typical group format. This presentation of an agenda is useful in orienting members to the session and is also designed to help reduce anxiety. One co-leader takes the lead in discussing the agenda, and the other participates by reinforcing, clarifying, or adding information as needed. The components of the first session's agenda that are included at this time are (1) the overview of the group's guidelines, (2) the "introductions exercise," (3) the initial goal statements, and (4) the "closing round."

Following their description of the first session's agenda, co-leaders provide members with psychoeducation about the normal weekly sessions and the overall structure and format of the therapy. They describe each typical session (check-in, sharing and feedback, closing round) as well as the process for the therapy over time (introductory phase, goal work, concluding phase). Co-leaders reinforce the importance of members' using external supports and taking good care of themselves, and help members to anticipate emotional challenges that they are likely to experience at some point during the therapy, especially when memories of trauma are shared. Members are offered the opportunity to ask any questions they may have before transitioning from the initial orientation to more specific content.

Description of Group Guidelines

Next, the co-leaders review the general guidelines for TRG treatment and pass out the summarizing handout (which is provided in Appendix F). Some key group guidelines include confidentiality, mutual respect, no out-of-group contacts with one another, and the policy on lateness and absences. The following information should be provided about these key guidelines:

Confidentiality

In order for group members to feel safe in sharing highly personal aspects of their lives and work on their goals, it is vital that everyone understand and respect the confidentiality of the group. It is acceptable for clients to discuss their experience of the group with their individual therapists, where confidentiality is observed. Beyond this boundary, while participants can of course choose with whom they wish to discuss their own therapeutic work, they may not speak about others and their experiences.

Mutual Respect

It is important that members interact with one another respectfully by listening and not interrupting one another. It is also important that members respect the boundaries of one another's time for sharing in the group. Disagreement is acceptable and indeed is often helpful, so long as it is managed respectfully.

No Out-of-Group Contacts

Contacts among members outside of the group sessions are actively discouraged. Such contacts can threaten the safety and productivity of the group in that they dilute the therapeutic value of material brought into the group, foster exclusive relationships among members, and introduce interpersonal dynamics that distract members from their goal focus. If group members happen to meet each other in another setting, members may politely acknowledge each other and perhaps engage in "small talk" unrelated to the group, but anything else should remain within the group. Some group members may prefer not to be acknowledged outside of the group, as the chance encounter may involve explaining to *someone else* how they know the other person. Members should be asked their preferences on out-of-a-group acknowledgement. Co-leaders should specify that they will not acknowledge members outside of the group's sessions unless the client initiates the contact. Members should be told that options for continued contacts with others after the group ends will be discussed during the concluding sessions.

No Touching of Others

For many people—especially victims of violence and abuse—being touched by someone else can seem like an invasion of one's personal space and be detrimental to one's sense of safety and trust. Although it is tempting for group members to console one another through touch (e.g., a hug, or hand on the back), it is important to encourage members to use words instead to express empathy or support.

No Food

While members may bring a beverage to group sessions, solid food is distracting and therefore not allowed.

Lateness and Absences

Group members should be informed that they are expected to attend regularly and arrive at each session on time. In the event that a member is going to be late or absent, she should let the group leaders know as soon as possible in advance so that this information can be communicated to the group. Clients should understand that inconsistent attendance is highly disruptive to the group and that members may become unduly concerned whenever someone does not show up for a session without an explanation or may misattribute it to something that they or someone else might have said within a prior session.

Next, group leaders should address members' questions about the foregoing material and elicit discussion about any other suggested guidelines that might help them feel more comfortable in the group. In addition, group members should be forewarned that at times the group experience might evoke strong feelings as they work on their trauma recovery. The key role self-care should be emphasized. At this juncture, group leaders begin to describe the ways in which they will interrupt or intervene with members during sessions to help keep them on task, adhere to a guideline, or assist in goal development. These interruptions and the active role of the group co-leaders during early sessions are framed as part of their role in keeping the group safe as well as facilitating overall work toward goal development and achievement.

There are often questions about the group guidelines, some of which reflect confusion or imply disappointment from members. The focus of these questions is frequently related to out-of-group contacts. Some sample questions or concerns and suggested responses are detailed below, and additional examples are provided in the "Common Challenges" section at the end of this chapter.

> GROUP MEMBER: I am so lonely. I think most trauma survivors are. I don't understand why we cannot be friends and support one another outside of the group. I thought the purpose of this group was to make connections.

> GROUP LEADER: We really do understand the loneliness and isolation that often result from having the painful and traumatizing life experiences you have all had. In addition, though, it is important that we pay the utmost attention to creating a safe experience for you and all group members. We have found that limiting out-of-group contact helps members to feel more secure about their relationships in the group without having to worry about feeling left out or struggling to be included in outside contacts. This guideline also helps to minimize the risks that can inadvertently arise around the issue of confidentiality when members start using each other for support outside of the group time. Each of you is in this group because *you all have additional supports in your life*. I hope this explanation helps. Over-

all, this group can definitely help to reduce your isolation, but we anticipate that will happen most safely emotionally within group time for now.

In this example, the client's concern provided an opportunity to integrate psychoeducation about the interpersonal impact of trauma with information about the rationale for specific boundaries within the group.

How to manage this guideline in practical terms is also often a source of initial confusion, as in this exchange:

GROUP MEMBER: So, do you mean we should just nod or sit silently in the waiting room or if we bump into each other somewhere? I need a little clarification on that.

GROUP LEADER: Good question. I am glad you asked, because what we are really striving for is safety and confidentiality. What we often find is that some members are most comfortable remaining quiet, acknowledging each other in a brief nonverbal way. Others may prefer to make small talk about the weather or something unrelated to the therapy. The two most important things to keep in mind are to respect each other's choices about how much chatting happens and to keep any chatting to minor nongroup-related topics.

Introductions Exercise

At this point in the first session, all group members participate in an "introductions exercise" in which group members each pair off with the person to her right and the two interview each other. Members are instructed not to talk about the details of their trauma history at this time but rather to inquire about each other's life in the present. This juncture is a very important moment for co-leaders to do a time check with each other. The amount of time designated for members to interview each other is partially determined by the remaining session time, as a round of goal check-in and a closing round are still to follow. These two remaining portions of the session can be expected to take about 20 minutes. A co-leader describes the introductions exercise as follows:

"Each of you is here today because you have been through trauma, but this is an opportunity to remind yourself and others that there is so much more to who you are. Think about sharing some information about yourself such as your hobbies and interests, your living arrangements, family, occupation, cultural or ethnic background, pets or a favorite animal—everybody has many things to share. You can choose to interview each other or just to interact as in a conversation. We [group leaders] will also participate in this exercise. We will let you know when we are about halfway through the interviewing time. Please feel free to find any place in the room where you feel most comfortable to talk."

The group leaders pair up with each other and converse about matters that they feel comfortable sharing with the group. After about 5 minutes (or the designated time), the pairs reconvene, and each person in turn takes a few minutes or sentences to introduce her partner. Before moving on to the next pair, the person being introduced is given an opportunity to add to or correct anything that has been said. The co-leaders usually model this process by first introducing each other. It is our belief that disclosures about a therapist's own trauma history are not appropriate at this time or at any other time during this group process, as such information tends to be a burdensome distraction. It may be useful, however, to share one's reasons for choosing to work with trauma survivors. Additional shared information should be focused on professional identity and perhaps a detail about a hobby, interest, or self-care activity.

During this introductory exercise the level of anxiety in the room usually begins to fall, as members gradually adjust to talking within the group setting and start to seek common ground with their peers. An example of how group members may introduce each other follows:

> SARA: This is Maria. She is from Kansas and now lives in Cambridge on her own. She has four children and two grandchildren whom she takes care of a few days a week. Her son is in the military and was stationed in Iraq, but he is now home safely. She used to work in retail but quit last year because she had some health problems. Oh—and she just got a puppy.

> MARIA: This is Sara. She is originally from Colombia but has lived in this country for many years. She has a sister who lives nearby. She teaches in a school for children with special needs. She enjoys doing art and learning about different religions.

> GROUP LEADER: Is there anything that was not mentioned that either of you would like to add?

> SARA: I think she covered everything.

> MARIA: I wanted to add that I heard this week that I was approved for disability, which is a huge relief.

> (*Group members congratulate Maria on this news.*)

At the end of this introductions exercise, group members are complimented for taking their first steps in sharing about themselves, and they are reminded that as the group develops they will get to know one another on many levels.

Initial Statement of Goals

The next agenda item during the first session is an initial goal statement by members. This activity facilitates the sharing of more personal information in a paced way and begins to set the stage for the goal focus that will be central to the structure and format of the overall group experience. Members are reminded that, prior to this session, they each identified a general area in their current lives in which they are aware of the impact of their trauma. They are asked to briefly share what they can about the formulation of their goal, which may range from a broad topic such as reducing isolation to a more specific action such as disclosing a secret related to the trauma to a family member or friend. Members are reminded that at this early stage there is no expectation of complete goal formulation, as the process of identifying and clarifying goals will take place over several weeks of therapy and the goal may change over time. Unlike future sessions, this process is handled in the style of a check-in rather than split between goal work and feedback. Occasionally group leaders will intervene to help a member focus or to offer guidance to a member as indicated by her comments. It is sometimes helpful to ask group members to repeat their name before speaking during this round. An example of this initial goal statement "go-around" follows (without the name repetition):

JESS: I haven't worked it all out yet, but I feel like I live a lot of my life with secrets from the world, and I want to change that. So, maybe the goal is about trust, or maybe something like that.

MARIA: I have a family wedding coming up, and some people who aren't safe for me will be there, but I really want to go for my cousin. I want to work on finding a way to deal with this. I guess I feel like that is kind of lame . . .

GROUP LEADER: Actually, it sounds very important that you are thinking ahead about your needs and recognizing risks. I think you will be able to formulate your goal more over time and that the group will be very helpful as you try to sort out the possibilities. And I hope over time you'll come to feel that you don't need to apologize for your goal—there's nothing lame about it!

MARIA: Thanks.

SUSANNA: I really struggle with goals; so, picking one and following through will be the art of my work, I guess. I don't really think about life in terms of accomplishments, because they seem like a set-up for disappointment. So, my joining this group— like for all of us—is a big deal. We are all so brave!

NANCY: I totally agree, Susanna. I have so many traumas that I can't decide which one to focus on for this group. I had an idea and then it changed. I guess I am more confused about my goal than I was at the intake. I think I need to move away from focusing on the traumas and look at my life now—as you said . . . but I hate to do that! Well, I guess I have my work cut out for me. I can't wait to have more help from the group!

SARA: I think I want to tell my mother about what my uncle did to me . . . the abuse . . . but I am not sure if that is a good idea or not. My therapist suggested that figuring out something about that could be a good group goal for me, and I agree.

LISA: Hmm. Even this is hard to say. Sometimes people tell me that I come across so differently from how I mean to. It can be a negative thing. I think it is because I am so disconnected from my feelings. So, there's that. I am also really isolated, so something about one of those areas will be my focus.

A group leader concludes this round with a summarizing statement about goal development and the preliminary scheduling of time taking for the next session. This statement includes some psychoeducation about common reactions to traumatic experiences, which is central to resolving the shame that many trauma survivors carry with them. The group leaders also address the importance of individual paths to recovery. This acknowledgment of diverse approaches to wellness helps to foster a new relational experience for the group members in which both individual and collective goals are valued. A group leader states at this point:

"Although each of you is in a different place around your goal development, you are all on your way. The themes of trust, isolation, disconnection, shame, and confusion that came up in your go-around are all common reactions to trauma, but the path of recovery, the goal you choose, and the process by which you achieve it will be unique to each of you. We want to encourage you all to use both group and your individual therapy as you embark on this process of goal development and achievement. In a moment we will move to the closing round. Next week we will begin our usual time sharing after we [the co-leaders] take some time to review that process. Are there two volunteers who are willing to begin to elaborate on their goal formation next week by providing some context and sharing further about where they are in goal development? You would talk for about 10 minutes, and then there would about 10 minutes of feedback from members to help you with your work. We will explain the process in more detail next week."

Typically, two or more volunteers will speak up. At this point, a tentative time sharing order for the upcoming weeks is established. If there are no volunteers, the group leaders (based on their judgment of who seems most ready) should ask two particular members to take time the following week.

Closing Round

During the closing round, group leaders should remind members that simply starting to participate in a trauma group can, in itself, be emotionally evocative, and the leaders should help them to anticipate that they may experience a worsening or resurgence of symptoms, at least initially. Before they depart, members are each asked to say a few words about how they are feeling and to share a self-care strategy that they instead to use after the session. For example:

SUSANNA: This was less scary than I thought it would be. I am going to eat a healthy dinner and watch some TV.

MARIA: I am glad that I am here, but I still feel nervous. I am going to take a long bath and call a friend.

NANCY: I am so busy, but now I am thinking and feeling a lot about this group. Self-care, hmm . . . I think I will let myself call a friend who makes me laugh before I return to working.

JESS: I am feeling a little floaty. I know I need to practice mindfulness on my way to the bus, and that will help. I also have some soothing music to listen to on the way home.

LISA: I am okay. This was not as bad as I thought it would be. I am going to get take-out food and watch a movie.

SARA: I feel good that I came—I thought I might chicken out on the way here! I am a little worried about finding a good goal, but I will talk about it with my therapist when we meet tomorrow. I am going to practice my guitar when I get home—that usually helps me to relax.

In the rare event that a member feels very distressed or is dissociated during the closing round, the group leaders should intervene (see the "Common Challenges" section at the end of this chapter for more details on how to address these issues). Otherwise, the group ends with a farewell from the leaders, who remain in the room as the members leave.

It is extremely important for co-leaders to take time immediately after the group session to review what occurred during the session and to write notes to be shared with the supervisor, using the form provided in Appendix G. Following this first session, the information to take to the supervisor will be more general than that outlined on the form; however, establishing this precedent will be especially helpful as the group continues (a completed example of Appendix G is included in Chapter 7 as Figure 7.1). In addition, co-leaders are referred to Appendix H as a means of keeping track of who will be "taking time," from week to week; a filled-in example is included as Figure 4.1. This tool will become particularly

---

Co-leaders complete this form outside of group time following Session 1 or 2 (and later on, as needed) when the order of participants' turn taking has been established. Cycle through the order repeatedly, with three clients taking time each week. If the group has fewer or more than six members, the use of this tool is especially important in eliminating confusion or error. It is also helpful in monitoring changes (e.g., if the cycle is disrupted by a group member's absence) and in keeping track of how many "turns" a client has left before the end of the therapy.

Week 1_____ (introductions, orientation)

No time taking.

Week 2_____ (only 2 time takers in Session 2)

Overview of new information

Member: Jan_____

Member: Melanie_____

Week 3_____

Member: Anna_____

Member: Lenore_____

Member: Pat_____

Week 4_____

Member: Susan_____

Member: Jan_____

Member: Melanie_____

. . . Repeat rotation through the concluding phase.

FIGURE 4.1. Time-taking tracking tool.

useful in keeping track of who will be sharing their goal work each week as group sessions unfold over the course of the treatment.

SESSION 2

The second session begins with establishing the norms for the "opening round," when everyone "checks in." The co-leaders remind the group that each member should simply state their names and "say a few words about how you are doing as we begin the group today." Following this check-in, the group leaders again acknowledge that it is a big step forward to participate in this kind of group and further normalize the fact that doing so may have stirred up some trauma-related memories and/or symptoms. They also honor the fact that everyone has returned after the initial session, or they explain any absences. Finally, they remind members that the first few sessions are somewhat atypical, departing from the usual agenda.

The co-leaders then briefly review what occurred during the preceding session (particularly the group guidelines) and provide an overview of what will be covered during this session.. Following the check-in and prior to members' time sharing, the co-leaders claim 20–25 minutes (replacing the time that would normally be claimed by one group member) to talk about individualized goals and the guidelines for sharing and giving feedback. These are discussed in detail below.

Individualized Goals

The co-leaders explain that the TRG's initial sessions are focused on goal formation. They describe the qualities that make for a well-conceived goal (i.e., that it be trauma-related, present-centered, realistic, concrete, and specific—see Chapter 2) and the collaborative process of setting, tracking, and renegotiating goals. This information will take on more meaning for members as they begin engaging in their work, and it will become incorporated in co-leader feedback in future sessions. This summary of how to individualize their goal is important, and it also represents an introduction that will warrant frequent and detailed repetition. This may be a propitious time to explain to group members that the co-leaders will be very active in helping members understand sharing, feedback, and goal development. Co-leaders end this discussion by answering any questions members have about the general topic of individualized goals.

Guidelines for Sharing and Feedback

The co-leaders next describe some general guidelines for sharing personal information and giving feedback (reviewed in detail in Chapter 2). In regard to sharing, they should highlight the importance of keeping focused on what is relevant to one's goal and of "checking in" with oneself while doing so. If members want a specific kind of feedback, they are encouraged to *ask* for what they want. Members should be encouraged to keep feedback relevant to the goal of the person who is sharing and focused on *her* experience. Making observations and asking questions are both potentially helpful ways of giving feedback. The co-leaders should assure the group that they will monitor and help direct sharing and feedback whenever necessary and that there is a learning process associated with these skills. Again, group members are then provided with an opportunity to ask any questions about sharing and giving feedback before moving on.

Common Questions and Concerns

The structured sharing and feedback components of the TRG model are unfamiliar to most clients, even (and sometimes *especially*) if they have participated in other types of psychotherapy or self-help groups. It thus can take a few sessions for members to start feeling comfortable with this style of interaction. At this early stage, some members may express uncertainty about how to know what information is relevant for sharing. A group leader might respond in the following way:

> "There are two helpful guidelines to keep in mind as you consider sharing information during your allotted time. First, it is very important to check in with yourself to see how you feel about sharing the information. Are you ready to do so or are you feeling disconnected or overwhelmed (which may suggest that you not share at that moment)? Second, it is important to ask yourself whether this information is relevant to your goal establishment or progress. There will be times when each of you has important things happening in your life that you would like to spend your time talking about but that are not related to your goal. In those moments, we will check in with you to help you to remain goal-focused."

Survivors of chronic interpersonal trauma often have difficulty regulating self-disclosure, tending either to hold back on sharing their experiences and feelings altogether or disclosing too much before they have established a sense of internal and relational safety. In responding as above, the group leader also goes on to draw attention to several guidelines that are important in preparing group members for the Stage 2 trauma work ahead. These include attention to pacing and timing, monitoring and modulating affect so that it is not too much or too little, and using the aforementioned goal focus to contain and control how much is disclosed and in what detail.

Another common concern about sharing is that group members worry about whether they will have enough to talk about during their allotted sharing time. Group leaders might respond by reassuring the member that they will help her use her time productively in explaining her goal work and that she need not worry about having to manage it alone. They may also reassure her that there is flexibility in regard to allocating time between sharing and feedback and that this division may vary somewhat, depending on the work she is doing in session.

In regard to feedback, a group member might be confused about asking questions, perhaps wondering whether her question was too intrusive or upsetting. The group member should be reassured that asking questions is a helpful form of feedback that enhances the collaborative aspect of goal formation and mutuality. This occasion might also be another opportunity to remind members that questions should always relate to the member who is sharing and her goal rather than the questioner. Group leaders should advise members to "check in with themselves" before sharing information, keep in mind that they are always in control of what they share and that this decision should be guided by their own affective response. Finally, leaders should often reiterate the importance of maintaining a respectful tone.

As another example, a group member may express concern about her tendency to want to help or take care of others by giving advice, thereby naming a way she imagines that feedback could be challenging for her. Group leaders may respond as follows:

> "It is a good first step that you are aware of this possible personal challenge for yourself. In general, it is more helpful to offer suggestions based on your own experience or thoughts rather than engaging in giving advice. This is a place and situation where we [the co-leaders] would step in to help you to frame your thoughts more effectively. We do not expect members to understand immediately the most helpful ways to give and receive feedback, but we will help you, and as the group progresses and you have more practice, your own judgment will also improve. You will all be learning this particular way of communicating in tandem with one another.

Group leaders should inform members that if they prefer a particular type of feedback (e.g., help in understanding a particular problem or how to deal with a specific situation, monitoring their connections with affect), they can ask for it directly. Members should also be told that the co-leaders will check in with them from time to time about whether they are receiving the kind of feedback that is helpful and will try to redirect the feedback process if that is not the case. This communication reinforces the message that group members' needs are respected as important and encourages members to express their own needs. By practicing self-expression in the safe relational context of group, members develop a skill that they can also practice in outside relationships.

Time Taking

The remainder of the session, except for the last 5 minutes (the closing round), is usually divided among the two members who volunteered to share at the end of the first session. The co-leaders should suggest that each group member use her time to let the group know where she is in regard to formulating her goal and how this goal is relevant to her present life. The leaders should caution that this is not the time for members to share detailed information about their histories of trauma, as they are just getting to know one another, and that there will be ample time for this kind of sharing in future sessions. Again, this communication conveys the idea that safe self-disclosure is gradually paced and should be preceded by getting to know others and establishing a sense of relational safety.

Approximately halfway through the allotted time period, the co-leaders should ask the person sharing whether she is ready to hear feedback from others. During the remainder of her time, group members and co-leaders ask questions and offer observations about what has been shared. Throughout the TRG, co-leaders should actively model empathetic feedback and invite others to join in this process. However, this is especially important during the initial phase—when all members may be more anxious and inhibited about speaking—to ensure that an individual's sharing is not met with repeated and prolonged silence.

Case Example 1

Belinda is an example of a client who came to the group with an out-of-group goal that was subject to further definition during her turn in the second session of the group. Belinda began by stating that her goal for the group was to feel less anxious around men. She disclosed that she had been sexually abused by her brother over several years and that she avoided dating in high school and college, immersing herself instead in her studies. She reported that as an adult she had had one relatively brief relationship with a man that ended when she found out that he was cheating on her. Belinda is employed in a managerial job in which she is successful, but she shared that she felt like a failure in her social life. She stated that her sisters and friends are all married or partnered, and that she feels lonely and set apart from them.

During feedback time, various group members identified with Belinda's fearfulness in regard to men. One member asked if Belinda felt anxious around all men, and she replied that her anxiety was especially pronounced in social situations (e.g., parties), where there was the possibility for romantic involvement. She elaborated that whenever she is approached by a man at a social gathering, her heart starts racing, she begins to panic, and she feels as though she must escape. Another member asked how Belinda typically deals with her anxiety; she responded that she usually either avoids such situations or makes an excuse and leaves. A co-leader asked how Belinda would like to be able to deal with such situations. She responded that she would like to be able to reduce her anxiety sufficiently so that she can remain in the situation long enough to determine whether a real threat to her safety exists. The other co-leader wondered about whether there was a way for Belinda to monitor her anxiety levels over the course of the group. Belinda stated that she had previously used subjective units of distress (SUDs) ratings in her individual therapy sessions and could use this technique to quantify how anxious she feels in social situations. At present, whenever she is in a social situation, her anxiety level reaches 9 or 10 on a scale of 0–10.

In this example, Belinda comes into group therapy with a fairly clear goal focus, but she needs the group's help to work toward more specificity. Group members' support and curiosity assisted Belinda in sharing more details about her experience. The co-leader was instrumental in introducing a way in which Belinda could measure her progress as she works toward diminishing her anxiety, which leads to avoidance.

Case Example 2

In the following example, the co-leaders helped Marta understand how to pace her sharing during this early stage of the TRG.

MARTA: Before I start, I just want to say that I am totally curious about why we are all here. Are we ever going to share about that . . . like about exactly what happened to us?

CO-LEADER 1: That is a good question and one that many of you may have. As part of your goal development, each of you will share what you want to about your history and why you are here. The amount of information that each of you shares will depend upon what is comfortable for you. For some, sharing your experience in a connected way may actually be the key goal you work on.

CO-LEADER 2: Try to remember that these are new relationships for all of you. We are just getting to know one another, and proceeding in a paced and careful way is very important.

MARTA: I really want to start by telling my story, if that is okay. I want to work on decreasing my isolation, and I just don't see that happening if people don't know about me and why I am here.

CO-LEADER 2: Before you start, I would like to ask a clarifying question. Could you say a bit more about what it would mean to you to decrease your isolation and how you see your isolation as being related to your trauma?

MARTA: Yes, I will do that as I tell you about my traumas. It will be pretty obvious.

CO-LEADER 1: Maybe you could start by describing the impact of your trauma on your current life, like how you feel isolated and what you might want to change, and then filling in the context with information about your trauma.

MARTA: Thanks, that's helpful. I tend to want to just dive in, and my therapist says that sometimes that scares people away. I don't want to scare you away . . .

CO-LEADER 1: I don't think you are likely to scare people away here, but this is a place where you could practice starting relationships a little differently as a part of your goal.

MARTA: Okay, good. I don't want to be sitting here in therapy thinking I am going to scare people away, but the way you put it makes sense to me. It's not about being scary here—it's about trying something different. So, let me just say the traumas in my life started before I really can even remember. I feel like they define who I am, so talking about myself without telling you all about them is really hard.

In the preceding vignette, the co-leaders intervene early and actively during the sharing session of the member's time, sensing that Marta is about to overdisclose, perhaps as a distraction from goal focus, or—as Marta is able to say—because she struggles to see herself as anybody but a trauma victim. Through gentle psychoeducational intervention, the leaders are able to help Marta understand reasons for pacing that differ from previous experiences where perhaps she has "scared people away." This interaction helps Marta to reframe her thinking and is observed by group members, who also benefit from the modeling of safe guidance.

Closing Round

The group concludes with a 5-minute closing round during which members state their feelings as they leave the group and identify a way in which they will nurture themselves after leaving the session. Group leaders remind members that those who did not "take time" this session will do so the following week.

SESSIONS 3–5

Session 3 marks the beginning of what will be the typical weekly session, in terms of the group process. Since members have a rudimentary familiarity with the group structure and guidelines discussed during the introductory sessions, time sharing constitutes almost the entire session (with the exception of the opening and closing rounds). Before members begin sharing, the co-leaders take a moment to divide up the time equally so that members are well aware of how much time they are allotted. Leaders take the primary responsibility for monitoring adherence to the schedule. The co-leaders explain that group members who did not take time the preceding week will have a turn in this session or the next to begin working on their goals. They are also reminded that subsequent sessions will follow this established sharing schedule whereby members take time to share in rotation.

Leaders make clear that, during the remaining sessions of the introductory phase, the primary task for each group member will be to finalize her goal so that it is operationally defined, related to her trauma history and its impact on her present life, and achievable within the time frame of the therapy. In addition to facilitating this process, co-leaders are attentive to the ongoing development of members' understanding of the structure, guidelines, and sharing/feedback components of the TRG. This task often requires that leaders be highly active until the group momentum becomes more self-sustaining through more clearly defined individual areas of focus and increased comfort with the essential attributes of the group culture.

If a member has a defined and workable goal, she should use this time to provide the group with more context and detail so that others can understand how this goal has come to be important in her life and how it is relevant to her trauma history. At this point, group leaders encourage members to provide a general sense of their background and history of trauma. The following extended case example illustrates the process of facilitating goal development during this stage of the group.

Case Example

Sarah is a 34-year-old professional sculptor. She is very driven in her career and has enjoyed creative productivity for most of her professional life. She comes to the group having experienced physical abuse in childhood by her mother and a rape 3 years ago after being drugged at a party. Since the rape, Sarah has been unable to produce art of any kind and has had to rely on income from temporary work, which has been a tremendous source of frustration for her. She reports that she feels "stuck" and as if she is "just existing." Her motivation for joining the group is to figure out how and why the rape has prevented her from accessing her creativity and to be able to begin sculpting again. Sarah disclosed the above information during her first turn to share, and now, during the fourth session, she expresses frustration that she is not feeling as though she is making progress.

Sarah begins her sharing time by restating her general goal focus and expressing frustration that she does not feel any more creative or hopeful than she did a week ago. At this point, a group leader intervenes and asks Sarah to elaborate a bit more on what she is expecting of herself on a weekly basis. Sarah responds that she feels like she is supposed to be able to notice changes every week and that all she notices is that she is feeling increasingly frustrated with her lack of productivity. Empathically acknowledging these feelings, the group leader normalizes this experience, noting that engaging in a process and trusting in an outcome can be very challenging for many trauma survivors, especially those who have relied on their accomplishments to feel okay about themselves. Sarah picks up on this point of psychoeducation and notes that she has heard this feedback before but that it has never made a difference in her life to know this. She also reiterates her impression that the idea of a goal implies ongoing noticeable progress for her, which is a major reason she misses being able to sculpt.

Although only about 8 of Sarah's designated 12 minutes of talking time have passed, given that she seems to be speaking about a highly salient aspect of her goal-focused experience, a co-leader interrupts and asks Sarah if she would be open to stopping at this point and hearing feedback from other group members. Sarah agrees. After a moment of silence, group members respond by expressing understanding of Sarah's frustration but also curiosity about the impact of her trauma on this experience. Sarah sits quietly, looking very sad. Another member observes the shift in Sarah's affect and offers the feedback that Sarah seems to understand something very important about the role of producing in her life.

Another member asks how the pressure to produce feels connected to her trauma history. Sarah thinks for a moment and responds that, in fact, one of the frequent excuses for her childhood beatings was that she was accused of being "lazy" and "useless" for not helping more around the house. One group member, Jan, relates to Sarah's experience of verbal abuse and begins to tell details of her own history. As this is Sarah's time, a group leader interrupts gently but firmly, acknowledging Jan's story but reminding her to focus her feedback on Sarah. Jan stops for a moment and shares that what she wanted Sarah to know is that she is not alone in this struggle and that maybe her early history is playing a bigger part in her struggle to produce than she had previously thought. This idea is echoed by other members, who are able to notice that Sarah seems to have developed a new understanding of her difficulty in producing art during her present circumstances. Sarah, although quiet, seems to be taking this feedback in, and she is observed to be nodding her head in agreement with what she is hearing. A co-leader asks her if she can speak to what she is feeling, but Sarah says she needs some time to think about this feedback, as she had thought that the difficulties she is having right now were primarily related to having been raped. A co-leader comments that experiencing trauma as an adult can reactivate feelings and reactions associated with even earlier trauma. She also says that Sarah is making progress toward refining her goal and that progress does not always come in expected ways. She suggests that Sarah may want to narrow her goal to allow herself more time to be in a process of understanding in regard to the impact of her childhood trauma on her current difficulty in sculpting. She adds that Sarah's goal of returning to sculpting remains important and that it ultimately may be more successfully accomplished if broken down into smaller steps.

Discussion

This example of early group process incorporates several common goal development themes and interventions of the TRG. First, as members are adjusting to the group's goal focus, feelings of frustration and self-criticism are not uncommon. This sense of turmoil provides an opportunity for a co-leader to intervene and offer psychoeducation that is likely to be helpful to many members of the group but is directly focused on Sarah, as it is her designated time period for sharing.

Given that Sarah responds with material that directly relates to her goal but does so with feelings of frustration, the co-leader decides to ask Sarah whether she is open to immediately hearing feedback, as supportive questions or comments from peers may help her with her expressed emotional bind. This kind of flexibility in the use of members' time occurs more frequently during the early phase of the therapy, reinforcing the collaborative process of goal development. Later on in the therapy, it is generally not helpful to ask for a sudden switch to feedback before most of a member's sharing time has been utilized. On very rare occasions, there may be a moment of feedback and a return to member sharing before formal feedback time begins. In all of these cases, the leader must be clear about holding the frame and naming the process. In addition, any changes outside of the allocated sharing and feedback time breakdown should be presented as a question to the member concerned whose time it is, and her response should be honored. This approach reinforces her sense of control and the notion that her needs and preferences are important.

As members begin to share feedback, co-leaders' roles involve actively maintaining goal development focus and facilitating supportive feedback. These processes will become more natural for members as the therapy progresses if they are actively facilitated during the early phase. In this example, a co-leader interrupts a member whose feedback is becoming less relevant to Sarah and more focused on herself. This skill of interrupting and redirecting takes practice and is helped by general reminders to group members to expect this type of guidance. Just as members are asked to be supportive, this is an opportunity for leaders to model empathic but direct feedback. Members are less likely to feel silenced or devalued if they are also reminded of other avenues of support for addressing content relevant to their own struggles, such as their own sharing time in group and their individual therapy.

Observations of members' body language and facial expressions can help to connect them with their experiences and are often productive in facilitating verbal expression or empathetic connection from members. Leaders can model sharing these observations, although as their comfort within the group grows, members are usually able to express curiosity about what they witness in an empathic manner.

Finally, suggestions for refining goals are incorporated into feedback from co-leaders. As indicated in the foregoing examples, co-leaders listen for emerging themes about the kinds of trauma-related problems that might be most salient for each member, and they ask questions and offer observations about ways in which these problems can be translated into goals that are both achievable and meaningful. In the latest example, it is quite possible that Sarah could achieve a goal related to sharing and deepening her understanding of the impact of her trauma on her current difficulty in sculpting. She may even be able to add a second goal that could include trying to sculpt again and sharing that experience with the group, following accomplishment of her newly revised goal. Actual productivity goals should be carefully monitored and adjusted to assure a group member's success and overall experience of mastery.

Ongoing collaboration among co-leaders, members, and outside treaters is essential in the process of defining and refining group goals. Group members should be encouraged to continue talking about goal definition in their individual therapy between group sessions. Group leaders should maintain contact with members' therapists so that the latter are informed about what their clients are working on in the group. This kind of contact enables treating clinicians to support clients' group work and provide a venue for discussing interpersonal issues and feelings that may arise in the group but cannot be sufficiently processed there due to the containing time limits and exclusive goal focus.

COMMON CHALLENGES

As in all groups, challenges—that is, unanticipated difficulties—will inevitably occur in the TRG. The unique structure of the group, although designed to provide predictability and safety, is sometimes a source of difficulty for members as they learn the group culture during the early phases of the therapy. Prototypical examples are provided to illustrate problems that may arise during the introductory sessions, followed by suggestions regarding potentially helpful interventions for each situation. It is of course impossible to anticipate every problem that can arise in a group of this nature, and the group leaders must thus be guided by their clinical judgment and experience and should use appropriate consultations.

Prolonged Check-In/Closing Round

Group members sometimes have difficulty in containing their check-in comments and will instead use this time as a "turn," going into in detail about the past week, disclosing feelings evoked by the preceding session, or introducing what they hope to talk about during this session or the next one. Alternatively, they may use the closing round to add to something they said during their time, give feedback to another member, or raise problems with the group structure or process. A group leader should gently interrupt the member and remind her of the purpose of the check-in/closing round in this manner: "Say a sentence or two about how you are feeling as you begin or end this session." She should validate the importance of what the group member is saying and suggest an alternative, such as talking about this issue during her next time for sharing or processing it further in her individual therapy. It is sometimes also helpful for the group leader to make a general empathic comment such as "It can be difficult to leave the session when things feel unfinished," or "It is hard to keep focused during the check-in when there are so many things going on in your daily life that you wish you could talk about."

Occasionally, during the opening or closing round, a group member may disclose that she is experiencing an increase in suicidal or self-harming ideation or otherwise feels unsafe. In such cases, the group leaders should try to contain the discussion as much as possible after determining that there are no immediate threats to the member's safety. They should then ask the member to meet with them at the end of the session so that they can talk with her further and help her to come up with a safety plan. It is important that other group members be aware that the co-leaders are attending to this person to reduce their worry about her safety. When group leaders meet with the individual after the session, they should aim to assess imminent risk, provide basic containment, and connect her with other treatment professionals and supports as needed (e.g., her therapist, the local hospital emergency room).

Difficulty in Focusing on a Goal

Some clients feel overwhelmed by many areas of their lives and have difficulty in narrowing their focus to a single goal. For example, during her first time to share, Katie talks about all the goals she is working on in her life, including taking better care of her health, making decisions about her job, dealing with her anxiety, and making changes in her family relationships. She talks about feeling stressed and burdened by these problems, all of which she feels are related to her trauma history in some way. A group leader responds as follows to increase the likelihood of a mastery experience by breaking up her goal work into more manageable pieces:

> "It sounds as though you have a number of different goals that you have been working on over time. Given that this is a 4-month group, I wonder if you could pick one or two that seem like they are most important to you right now. . . . Maybe it would help to prioritize what to work on in this group if you were to think about which goals feel most connected to your experience of trauma."

Katie proceeds to talk about her difficulty in trusting people as a result of her history of childhood sexual abuse, and she goes on to describe how her anxieties about dangers in the world affected her past parenting and present relationship with her children. She identifies this area of her life as the one on which she wants to develop a goal for the group.

Goal Is Too General

Clients often require considerable assistance from group leaders in translating their goals from general ideas to specific plans. For example, Karen initially identifies working on her trust difficulties in relationships as her group goal, making a general connection between these problems and her history of abuse and abandonment. A co-leader validates the importance of this overall goal in her recovery and notes that many group members can probably identify with this problem. She points out, however, that the TRG is a short-term group and that it is important that Karen experience success in achieving her goal. She encourages Karen to break down the overall goal and make it more specific so that she could work on a piece of it during the therapy. The group leaders and members ask Karen questions about how her trust difficulties affect her present relationships and whether these difficulties are specific to particular kinds of relationships. Karen responds that her trust difficulties are most pronounced in hierarchical relationships and identifies her current relationship with her employer as a relevant example. Thus, with the help of the group, Karen shifts from focusing on a very general goal to one that references current difficulties in a particular relationship. As her group work continues, Karen will speak further about the specific problems that she encounters in this relationship, how they are reflective of a more general relational pattern, and how they are connected with her trauma history.

Sharing Too Many Trauma Details Early in the Therapy

Clients frequently come to a group of this kind with much apprehension about speaking about their trauma. Some may be believe that "getting it all out" as early possible will provide relief or that they cannot be understood or helped by the group unless all is known about what they suffered. However, it has been our experience that bringing such affectively charged material into the group setting before a sense of safety is established can be overwhelming and destabilizing for both the individual sharing and the other group members. The group is also intentionally designed to provide a relational model in which the development of safety and trust precedes intimate sharing. As noted earlier, this information should be conveyed to members by the group leaders in a preemptive psychoeducational way. However, despite overt instructions to avoid sharing too much detail about trauma histories during the initial sessions, it sometimes happens that a group member starts disclosing these details while talking about her goal or providing context.

In such cases, the group leaders should intervene gently but firmly and promptly, validating the importance of the experience that the group member is beginning to share and reassuring her that there will be time to speak about these details over the course of the therapy. The importance of pacing and developing comfort when engaging in trauma recovery work in the group should be reiterated, and the member should be reoriented to the task of defining her goal and providing some general context for its importance.

Difficulty in Giving Empathic Feedback

A sense of mutual support and understanding usually develops very quickly in TRG therapy. However, it is worth remembering that group members frequently have some deficits in their relational skills based on their histories of complex trauma. As a result, empathic failures will occur, particularly during the earliest phase of treatment before members have a practiced firsthand experience of what is and is not helpful in regard to providing feedback. For example, during her sharing time, Lisa provides some context for her goal by referring to her history of severe emotional neglect by her parents. During the feedback time, Karen asks, "Do you mean that there was no trauma in your childhood?"

In such situations, it is important that group leaders intervene quickly to redirect the feedback. In the present example, the group leader comments on how alone and unacknowledged the member must have felt as a child, and makes some psychoeducational statements about the painful long-term impact of emotional neglect. This feedback is validated by other group members depending on their experiences. Lisa goes on to say that she has blamed herself for the problems she experienced later on because she could see no major abuse in her childhood. In other instances, group leaders may need to model rewording or reframing a piece of feedback to convey a less judgmental tone.

Feedback Is Too Self-Referential

During the earliest phase of the therapy, it sometimes happens that members confuse "relating" to the experience of another client with providing feedback. For example, during her turn, Nancy apologizes for crying while telling her story, stating that she wishes she were stronger and did not allow her history to affect her so much. Susan responds that she is older than Nancy and has been in therapy for a long time but that she still cannot tell her story without sobbing. She goes on to describe in some detail various situations in which she has been overcome with tears, what this feels like, and how long it takes her to recover.

Once it becomes evident that a member has shifted from attending to the experience of the person sharing to focusing on her own experience, it is important that group leaders intervene gently but promptly to redirect the feedback. In this example, a group leader interrupts Susan respectfully, noting that it sounds as though she can really relate to how emotionally wrought Nancy feels when she speaks about her history. The leader reminds members about the guideline to keep feedback focused on the person who is sharing and asks Susan if there is a particular message that she would like to convey to Nancy based on her experience. Susan goes on to say that she wants Nancy to know that she is not alone and that she should not feel ashamed of her reaction. If Susan were to continue to use Nancy's time to process her own reactions, the group leader should intervene again, noting that this sounds like an important issue for Susan and suggesting that she talk about it further either during her next turn in the sessions or in her individual therapy.

Increased Symptoms during Initial Sessions

It is not unusual for members to report experiencing more psychological and physical symptoms during the early sessions of the group. Even though these sessions are carefully paced, members may be distressed by thinking and talking about their own past experiences as well as hearing about the stories of others. At this stage, members sometimes complain that there is insufficient closure at the end of the sessions and that they leave with painful feelings or with worries about others in the group.

It is important that group leaders normalize these predictable reactions in the context of participating in a trauma-focused group. At the same time, they should emphasize the importance of increased self-care and using available supports for the duration of the group. It may also be helpful to provide some brief psychoeducation about PTSD and other trauma symptoms. Group leaders should acknowledge how hard it can be to leave the session after painful feelings have been stirred up in oneself or others, but they should also convey a sense of confidence that members have the requisite coping skills and supports for dealing with these feelings. It is always important to preserve sufficient time for the closing round that members never feel that they are being rushed out of the room.

A Group Member Is Not Participating

It is expected that when a member is not actively sharing, she is engaged in listening and providing feedback. While it is not necessary for each member to provide feedback to every- one, it is important for the co-leaders to be aware if a member is silent for large segments of the session. It is generally not a good idea to call specifically on a member who has been silent. Instead, at an appropriate moment between "turns," it may be helpful for a co-leader to take note of a member's silence, gently providing her with an opportunity to clarify its cause (e.g., is she feeling preoccupied, dissociated, or angry?). A decision can then be made about what might be most helpful in reengaging her participation. For example, would it help for her to take some sharing time immediately even if she was not originally intending to do so? Although it is important to preserve the overall predictability and fairness of time sharing, it is certainly acceptable to reorganize turns from time to time in response to the particular needs of members. Often, however, simply making an empathetic observation about a member's silence can be helpful in enabling her to reengage in the feedback.

A Group Member Drops Out

Dropout rates for the TRG group tend to be low, given the rigorous screening process and typically rapid development of cohesion. However, it does sometimes happen that a group member leaves after only one or two sessions. For example, after attending the first session in which she is an active participant, Jean does not show up for the second session. When she is contacted by a group leader, she discloses that her abusive ex-husband, who had been living out of state for the past 2 years, recently returned and announced that he planned to seek custody of their two children. Jean reports that her symptoms have since become much harder to manage. Jean and the group leader agree that this is not a good time for her to participate in a trauma-focused group, as she needs to preserve her emotional resources to deal with the immediate crisis. The group leader follows up with Jean's individual therapist to inform her of this outcome.

In letting the group know about changes in membership, it is usually helpful to provide a brief explanation about why a member has left. Group leaders should ask the member who is leaving what she would like them to convey to the group about her departure. Once this information has been conveyed to the group, it is recommended that co-leaders provide a brief opportunity for members to voice their feelings and reactions. In this example, Jean indicated that she would be comfortable letting the group know that she was facing a legal case involving her ex-husband and that this had not been anticipated when she made her commitment to the group. She also asked the group leaders to let the other group members know that she enjoyed meeting them and to thank them for the kindness that she received during the sessions she attended. The group members expressed disappointment that Jean would not be participating further in the group.

CONCLUSION

The key elements of the TRG (focus on trauma, a set time limit, the goal orientation, time-sharing structure, supportive process, co-leadership) all begin to develop and accumulate significance during the early phase of the therapy. Members begin to disclose aspects of their trauma histories and the ways in which they believe their trauma has affected the area of their lives they are choosing to work on in the group. This gradual sharing is done with attention to both safety and affective connection, in preparation for the more sustained trauma focus that usually occurs during the next phase. Members begin to know one another, learn and use the group structure, and focus on the development of their goals. Members and co-leaders work collaboratively to implement useful guidelines for time sharing, and the goal focus becomes a source of personal growth and relationship building within the group. Psychoeducation is integrated throughout these processes as a tool to orient members to the group culture as well to provide valuable information directly influencing goal development and the recovery process. Consultation and supervision along with co-leader communication help to ensure that members and leaders maintain clarity about the overall process, which is directed toward goal development and achievement. The groundwork is set during the early phase of treatment for a fruitful healing experience for all members that is continued in the middle (goal-work) phase of the therapy, which we discuss next.

CHAPTER 5

Goal-Work Sessions

Typically, by Session 6 or 7 of the TRG, most group members will have formulated and refined their goals sufficiently to move into the next phase, which involves actively working on these goals within and/or outside of the sessions. Often this transition seems to occur organically, but usually group leaders should take note that the group is moving into a phase in which members start working on their goals. It is always helpful to remind members whenever the midpoint of the therapy has been reached. It has been our experience that reminding members of the time limit helps to spur action toward achieving the goals that they have set for themselves. We also recommend checking in with each client's individual therapist around this time. Often by sessions 10–12 various members will start to report having accomplished their goals. As these successes are welcomed with compliments, congratulations, and even applause within the group, frequently they set off a "chain reaction," prompting others to work more actively on achieving their goals.

During this phase of goal work co-leaders maintain the focus of the group by ensuring that the material that is processed is both *goal-relevant* and *trauma-related*. We strongly recommend that each member begin her turn in sharing by restating her goal, to encourage both more relevant sharing and more targeted feedback from others that in turn helps create the kind of goal mastery that is critically important for a group of this kind. During both the sharing and feedback portions of each member's turn, the co-leaders should be asking themselves (1) How is what is being spoken about related to this person's goal? and (2) How is what is being spoken about related to this person's trauma history? If the answer to either of these questions is unclear, the co-leaders should find a way of bringing it to the attention of the member and the group. While the manner of doing so will depend on the co-leaders' personal style, it is crucial to keep this frame of reference in mind or else the group may devolve into a support group and lose its emphasis on the mastery of past trauma. This issue is addressed further in the "Common Challenges" section at the end of this chapter.

It is especially important during this phase that group leaders rely on the use of the treatment's time-frame boundaries. By keeping close track of members' use of time, co-leaders contribute to the sense of safety developing within the group, help members better regulate their sharing by taking time into consideration as a form of self-care, and avoid problems associated with real or perceived inequities in time allotments. Clinicians find their own way of maintaining this type of structure. Whatever the style of management may be, however, group leaders should expect occasional challenges in their implementation of the schedule, as members delve more deeply into their goal work. Difficulties with time management require discussion between co-leaders and the supervisor as soon as they are noticed so that predictability can be maintained within the group. This need is discussed in greater detail in the "Common Challenges" section at the end of this chapter.

It is during this middle phase of the TRG that its Stage 2 trauma focus is most salient. As noted by Herman (1992b) and elaborated in Chapter 2, the work at this stage of recovery involves reconstructing the story, transforming traumatic memories, and mourning losses associated with the trauma. It is to be expected that group members will become very emotional during these group sessions as they recall and process traumatic memories relevant to their goal work and are confronted with inevitable losses that they experienced. In general, it is important for group leaders to be aware of the range of affect tolerance, both for each individual group member and for the group as a whole. Too little expression of feeling in the group leads to a collective sense of numbing and deadness; on the other hand, too extreme an expression of feeling creates a sense that the group is unsafe. As discussed in Chapter 2, group leaders should strive to conduct the group in a middle range of affective expression so that members feel fully engaged emotionally and moved but not frightened by one another. This attention to the "therapeutic window" (Briere, 1996) is a crucial aspect of successful Stage 2 work. By focusing consistently on goal work, group leaders can create a level of emotional intensity that is enlivening, but at the same time well-regulated and contained. Examples of how group leaders establish this balance are discussed later in this chapter.

Since the content of this phase of the therapy will vary widely, depending on the specific goals of each member, the remainder of this chapter addresses some general themes and some common challenges that may be expected to arise during this middle phase of the group treatment.

PROCESSING THE TRAUMA NARRATIVE IN A RELATIONAL CONTEXT

Disclosure of traumatic memories is a key component of working on the goals selected by clients in the TRG group and is a hallmark of Stage 2 trauma work in general. Indeed, any appropriate goal must be trauma-related in order to provide an avenue for structured exploration of traumatic experiences and their effects. The goal provides a context for disclosure and a means of keeping it relevant to the client's current life so that there is a real purpose for retelling trauma details. For example, a client with an in-group goal of being able to think and talk about her trauma story without dissociating would be encouraged to use her group time during this phase to speak about her trauma in a gradual and carefully paced way, monitoring her reactions both to her own telling and to the responses of others. A client might choose to take an initial step toward disclosing her abuse history to a family member or significant other by first sharing the events she will disclose to the TRG. A member might seek to understand a current difficulty in interacting with her employer by first exploring within the groups its origins in abusive encounters involving an authority figure in childhood. In the latter example, although telling the trauma narrative is not the ultimate goal, it is an essential step toward increased understanding of the behavior in question and having a greater range of choices in the present. For many clients, empowerment is born of the enhanced ability to differentiate between the residue of the past and present realities and to make decisions based on this new perspective.

The examples cited all involve telling some part of the trauma narrative. Members typically report considerable relief upon doing so, although the process itself frequently involves a temporary increase in symptomatology. As was noted in Chapter 3, we place great importance on careful pregroup screening so that temporary symptom exacerbation does not overwhelm members' coping.

In order for narrative sharing to be effective, it is crucial, first, that the member remain affectively connected with her own experience during the telling and, second, that the member feel connected with the group and be able to receive feedback. Group leaders can help the member remain affectively engaged with her narrative by asking questions about her feelings and gently noting their presence or absence in her nonverbal presentation, providing a model for group members to do the same. This approach often results in the member's accessing a variety of emotions associated with her experience of the trauma. Here it is really important to pay attention to pacing and to be checking in with the member about how she is feeling, asking whether she would like to continue or whether this would be a good time to stop for feedback.

The feedback segment of a member's time is an essential component of the group experience, further emphasizing the importance of effective time management. Members frequently are very anxious about what others are thinking during their sharing, anticipating that they will be judged. As has already been noted, it is important that the group leaders be active in modeling empathic feedback and inviting others to join. Another important aspect of the group leaders' role is to make sure that the member is able to "hear" the feedback. This requirement is sometimes accomplished by asking the member to repeat something that has been said and/or by asking her to reflect on how she feels when she hears this feedback. It is often useful to encourage the member to look at the person giving the feedback as well as the others in the room so that she can register not only the words that are expressed but also the nonverbal communications of empathy and support. It is not uncommon for a member to say that it is hard to believe compassionate feedback or that other members are "just being nice." Such reactions are usually challenged far more effectively by group members themselves than by the co-leaders. The integration of empathic feedback from the group is key to transforming trauma memories as this feedback directly contradicts the negative messages conveyed by abusers and the negative self-statements internalized by the client. The dissonance produced by this feedback—so long as the client is able to take it in—promotes favorable changes in group members' long-held beliefs about self and others.

Case Example 1: Mary

During the TRG's introductory sessions, Mary reports that she is consumed by feelings of shame and self-blame in response to memories of childhood sexual abuse by her uncle. She states that she knows intellectually that she was not responsible for the abuse but that she has difficulty in believing that this is true at an affective level. She identifies her goal for the group as transforming her feelings of shame and self-blame, and she indicates that she would know if she had made progress toward this goal if she were able to tell her story and experience some compassion for herself. With a great deal of anticipatory anxiety, Mary uses her time during this phase of the therapy to describe her memories of the abusive incidents. For the sake of Mary and the group, the co-leaders initially have to intervene to slow down the pace of the telling, as Mary acknowledges a desire to "get it over and done with." As Mary tells her story in a more emotionally connected way, it becomes apparent that much of her self-blame is rooted in statements made by the perpetrator during the abuse. For example, she recalls him telling her that they both were "damned" and would go to hell for what they had done. During the feedback, group members comment on the powerful impact of such words in shaping Mary's self-blame and in leading her to feel identified with the perpetrator as though she were an equal participant in the abuse. The group leaders validate the members' perceptions by commenting on the impact of the verbal and psychological abuse. Specifically, they refer to increasing evidence that verbal, emotional, and psychological abuse can be as pernicious as, or even more destructive than, other forms of abuse, particularly on survivors' sense of self and feelings of shame. During her next turn to share, Mary takes another risk and discloses that one of the most "shameful" aspects of her experience is her memory of feeling sexually aroused during the abuse. Several group members acknowledge being able to relate to this disclosure, which the group leaders immediately normalize by pointing out that the fact that her body was responsive to stimulation makes the experience no less abusive. Mary expresses great relief at receiving this feedback and not encountering the negative judgment that she had anticipated. She refers to this moment several times during subsequent sessions as a turning point in her work toward being kinder to herself. This example illustrates how, when a client experiences acceptance from other group members who bear witness her story (particularly after sharing aspects of it that she considers particularly shameful), her negative views of herself are challenged and ultimately may shift to a more compassionate self-stance.

In addition to providing a source of disconfirming evidence for challenging and transforming beliefs about self and others shaped by trauma, the connection that each member develops with the group as a whole helps to sustain her as she begins to mourn the losses associated with these experiences. Although the group support cannot take away the inevitable pain, the individual is reminded that she does not have to bear it alone and that others believe that she will ultimately be able to emerge from it and move on with her life.

Case Example 2: Stephanie

Stephanie, the single mother of a 4-year-old girl, came to the group complaining of difficulties in determining an appropriate level of protectiveness in relation to her daughter.

Stephanie, whose own mother had been an alcoholic and had been very neglectful, had experienced sexual abuse in early childhood by multiple perpetrators including her mother's boyfriend, a camp counselor, and the family physician. During the early sessions of the therapy, Stephanie spoke about wanting to protect her daughter from the very real dangers that exist in the world but at the same time worrying that by shielding her daughter in this way she was making her extremely anxious and not providing her with sufficient opportunities to explore and develop. She identified her goal as being able to arrange play dates for her daughter and to enroll her in a preschool program without experienced paralyzing anxiety about her safety.

During the goal-work phase, Stephanie spoke about her experiences of abuse by the multiple men into whose care her mother had entrusted her. She reflected on how her childhood might have been different had she not been traumatized in these ways, in the process accessing intense feelings of sadness and grief for the little girl that she had been. She described tearfully how this sense of loss tinges even her most loving and happy feelings toward her daughter. She spoke with great emotion about her observations from looking at old family photographs at how, as she got older, she appeared progressively less happy and more dissociated. She also expressed strong feelings of anger toward the men who had perpetrated the abuse and more significantly toward her mother, whom she felt had betrayed her by failing to protect her from the abuse. The group members listened attentively to Stephanie's recounting of her experiences and feelings. Members expressed their own sense of sadness about the losses of her childhood as well as their anger about the ways in which she had been hurt and abandoned. They also remarked about how painful it could feel to imagine what one's life could have been, had it not been so impacted by these experiences. The group leaders spoke about how trauma can influence parenting and beliefs about safety and also noted that survivors sometimes experience a resurgence or exacerbation of trauma symptoms when their child is at the age at which they were abused. Group members gently pointed out that the past could not be undone but that Stephanie had an opportunity to "set things right" in parenting her daughter. Members who had struggled with similar conflicts when their children were young shared strategies that they had used to make more objective decisions about safety. Hearing them talk in this way provided Stephanie with a sense of confidence that it was possible for her to learn how to be appropriately protective of her daughter while also fostering her development. She came up with some concrete ideas of her own about how to reduce her anxiety (e.g., by accompanying her child on play dates until she feels comfortable with other families; or talking with other parents whose children are currently enrolled in the preschool program about their experiences).

ORIENTATION TOWARD ACTION IN THE PRESENT

The exploration and processing of trauma memories in the TRG occurs in the service of working on present-oriented goals. In this goal-work phase of the TRG, members with in-group goals start trying out new behaviors in the group (e.g., talking about an aspect of their trauma that they have previously avoided, or working on remaining "present" while talking about their trauma). Members with out-of-group goals start taking steps toward doing something different in their lives outside of the group, using their time in the group sessions to reflect upon this experience and get support from others. Often this process involves confronting a situation that has been avoided owing to its connection with the trauma, such as setting limits in important relationships or disclosing the abuse to a family member or significant other. Group members can use their time for sharing and feedback to prepare for their out-of-session work, anticipating potential difficulties or reactions from others. In some instances, role play may be helpful in this preparation. Drafting a letter is another useful exercise, particularly for preparing a confrontation or disclosure. The draft letter is read aloud to the group, allowing for discussion and feedback. The group member may then choose whether or not to revise the letter and whether or not to send it.

Group members can also use their time to report back on the actions that they have taken and to process the emotional impact of their actions. Additionally, they can have an important "cheerleading" role, recognizing the hard work involved in implementing change and encouraging members to continue along this path. It is important for group leaders to acknowledge whenever a member takes major steps toward realizing her goal, as it may be hard for the person closes to the goal to see progress for herself.

Case Example 3: Lisa

Lisa came to the group with the goal of disclosing to her sister her childhood abuse by their father. During the introductory phase, she reported that she had been sexually abused by her father from the age of 3 until puberty. She believed that her mother had been aware of the abuse and that she had avoided addressing this issue with her mother directly to avoid painful feelings associated with this profound betrayal. She had one younger sister whom she had initially felt that she had protected by enduring the abuse. Later, she yearned to tell her but feared being disbelieved or ruining the seemingly close relationship that her sister had with her father. Spurred by concerns about the safety of her sister's young daughter, Lisa felt that the time had come to tell her sister about the abuse. Her ultimate goal of disclosing the abuse to her sister was initially "broken down" by co-leaders, who suggested that she start by speaking about her experience within the group as a step toward breaking the silence with her sister. As she did so and received the group's empathetic and validating feedback, she began to express a readiness to approach her sister. During the sessions preceding her visit to her sister, Lisa rehearsed how she might begin this conversation. With the help of the group, she identified some of her fears in regard to her sister's reaction and imagined how she might deal with these "worst-case scenarios." One of the ideas generated by the group was for her to stay at a hotel rather than at her sister's home in the event that her disclosure was received poorly and she needed a safe place to go. Lisa returned to the group reporting that her sister had not been as shocked as she had expected; in fact, she disclosed that she had recently been experiencing some vague memories of being inappropriately touched by their father. She expressed sadness on Lisa's behalf and guilt about how she had suffered, and the two began a discussion about confronting their mother. Lisa reported feeling empowered by having taken this step in disclosing to her sister—but also sad and angry that she might not have been able to protect her in the way she had hoped. The group and co-leaders provided feedback recognizing Lisa's courage in disclosing to her sister.

INCREASED GROUP COHESION

Given the rather homogeneous composition of the TRG, its goal focus, and its time-limited nature, there is typically a rapid development of a strong sense of cohesion. As members begin to share very personal aspects of their history and discover their commonalities, a sense of mutual understanding develops that inclines members toward greater intimacy and self-disclosure. In some groups, members occasionally share artwork or writings that express something important about them. During this phase of the therapy, it is also common for members to report feeling as though they are "carrying the group with them," as it were, between the sessions. In some cases, members may feel accountable to the group in regard to being active in pursuing the goals that they have set for themselves. In other cases, members may rely on their internal representation of the group to help them through a particularly challenging situation.

Case Example 4: Cathy

Cathy uses some of her group time to prepare for an upcoming family wedding that will also be attended by her abusive ex-husband. Although she does not anticipate feeling physically threatened by him, she worries about how she might react emotionally to his presence and how this might affect her ability to be involved in the wedding. As part of their feedback to Cathy, group members suggest various actions she might take to manage her anxiety, such as confiding her feelings to a cousin who knows about the abuse, asking not be seated near her ex-husband, and formulating an "escape plan" in case she needs to remove herself from the situation. When she returns from the wedding, Cathy proudly reports that although she felt anxious at times she was able to manage her feelings without needing to escape and she enjoyed reconnecting with family members whom she had avoided for several years because of their association with her ex-husband. She reports that she thought about the group feedback often over the weekend and drew strength from imagining the group members standing behind her.

INCREASED POTENTIAL FOR INTERPERSONAL CONFLICT

Almost paradoxically, as members begin to feel safer and more comfortable in the group, they may begin to take greater interpersonal risks as they try out new behaviors, creating the potential for conflict. Although interpersonal process is not the focus of the TRG, it arises inevitably in any group situation. It is therefore very important that the co-leaders have a good understanding of group dynamics. The decisions that group leaders make about how to respond to and utilize interpersonal conflict can determine whether it is ultimately helpful or a hindrance to the work of the group. In many cases, interpersonal conflict can be related to members' goals, and as such it can provide an extremely powerful opportunity in the here and now for the development of new insights and behaviors.

Case Example 5: Nancy

Nancy comes to the group complaining of difficulties in sustaining friendships. She elaborates that, while she is able to form relationships, she withdraws immediately if she feels hurt or criticized. Nancy shares her story of a long marriage to an alcoholic and violent husband. As the mother of three young children, she reports that she endured many beatings, partly because of her well-founded fear of what her husband might do to her if she tried to escape, but partly also because of her belief that "children need a father." She reports that she has become isolated from her former friends and has also become estranged from her sister, to whom she used to be close, because her sister has made remarks that Nancy interpreted as judgmental.

During feedback time, Martha, another group member, comments that she can't understand how anyone could put up with being so mistreated for so long. Nancy is deeply offended by this comment. She says she now feels "unsafe" in the group and threatens to leave. Martha tries to explain that she did not mean this as a criticism but rather as an awkward way of expressing sympathy. The other group members try to mediate, expressing support for Nancy but also affirming their belief that Martha meant no harm by her feedback. Nancy is unwilling to accept Martha's apology. She attends the next two group meetings but does not participate actively.

Since the problem seems insurmountable, the co-leaders schedule an individual meeting with Nancy. During this meeting Nancy acknowledges that she occasionally experiences an urge to flee or cut off relations with people in real-life situations in which she has felt disbelieved or invalidated and that this inclination has contributed to her isolation. She also acknowledges that she is so tormented by shame that she may have difficulty in distinguishing between a maliciously critical remark and one that might be insensitive but well intentioned. The co-leaders support this insight and discuss with Nancy how this situation might represent an opportunity to achieve some mastery over this repeated problem. Nancy agrees that simply staying in the group and being open to additional feedback might be a significant accomplishment. She is able to return to the group and share this insight without pursuing the conflict any further.

Most often, interpersonal conflict in the TRG is fairly limited and successfully processed in terms of its relevance to members' goals. Occasionally, however, the group's leaders are unable to defuse the conflict, or it becomes broader than can be dealt with through the member's goal-related work. In such instances, the leaders should acknowledge the conflict but also define clearly the parameters of what can be addressed in this particular group. They should encourage members to take unaddressed or unresolvable issues to their individual therapy sessions for further discussion and processing. In rare instances, it may be necessary for group leaders to meet individually with one or more group members involved in a particular conflict to determine how the member(s) can make the best use of the TRG if the conflict remains unresolved.

THE EVOLUTION OF GOALS: CASE EXAMPLE FROM A TRANSCRIPT

Among the most creative and demanding tasks for group leaders are maintaining a constant awareness of how individual group members are progressing toward their goals and taking an active role in helping group members shape their goals so that they move toward sharing the relevant trauma story in the group and toward taking specific needed actions. This process is both dynamic and collaborative. The group leaders help clients learn the process of "breaking down" their larger goals into more manageable and achievable steps. The member can then select one or more concrete steps that she can take in striving to accomplish her goal. In addition to increasing the likelihood that her goal will be achieved, one of the important advantages of approaching goal development in this way is that the member can leave the group feeling as though she has made some tangible progress toward furthering her goal even if it is not fully realized. Group leaders can help members "break down" goals by asking them to identify the various behaviors or concrete actions that might need to be implemented in order to feel that one has achieved the larger goal. Group leaders can help members prioritize and sequence these "subgoals" by asking them which specific behaviors or actions would be hardest to accomplish and which would feel most substantial once accomplished. In narrowing and refining goals, it is also often helpful to ask clients to imagine how they would feel in taking each of these steps and what impact its realization would have on themselves and their relationships. The more that group leaders model this type of engagement, the more that group members also become adept at helping one another deepen their understanding of their goals.

The case of Lenore illustrates how a goal may progress over the course of group therapy from a vague concept to a clear-cut action. When Lenore presents her goal for the first time, in the third group session, she states that she wants to "feel connected" to the group. This kind of feeling-state goal is not uncommon, reflecting the general sense of shame, isolation, and insecure attachment and numbness that afflict so many trauma survivors. The group leaders share this information with Lenore and the other members through a framing psychoeducational comment that helps to normalize Lenore's experience. In this early group session, the group leaders help Lenore define her goal in terms of some observable action by asking her how she would know if she felt connected. Through this process, her goal gradually evolves from a simple subjective feeling state to an interactive relational goal of being able to accept empathetic feedback without dismissing it. Lenore describes her goal as follows:

> "My problem is I keep people at a distance—I am really good at shrugging things off! I am really good at making other people feel comfortable and taking the focus off of me, and it is really hard for me to get down to the down and dirty of what is going on for me.

I could know people for years and still feel like they don't care about me! I feel really alone a lot, and most of the time, I like it that way. I also feel superior most of the time, not inferior. So, that sort of makes it okay for me to feel disconnected that way. But the truth is I always have that feeling of not being lovable and not feeling connected. So, my goal is that I would like to feel connected to this group. That is my goal."

The group leaders then ask for clarifications as an initial way of concretizing the goal, and invite feedback from other group members. They also call attention to the way that Lenore ignores positive feedback.

> GROUP LEADER 1: One question I have is: How would you know if you felt connected to the group? Is there any kind of sense of how you would know that?

> LENORE: I guess a couple things for me: I need to feel people "get it"—really get it! I never felt that people got it. And that includes my parents. I was always different, always the problem kid . . . But . . . actually, I don't know.

> GROUP LEADER 2: Do you feel open, at this point, to hearing feedback from people?

> LENORE: Yeah, very open to hearing feedback, and I am really anxious about being here—but I am also really happy to be here.

> SARAH: Well, I have to say that what you just did there is one of the gutsiest things that I have ever witnessed! You are so honest!

> LENORE: I really want this to change. It feels like the key. I don't want to live the rest of my life feeling this way. I am going to do whatever it takes to get there.

> GROUP LEADER 1: Were you aware of having an emotional or thought reaction when Sarah said that you were gutsy?

> LENORE: No.

> JOANNE: As you were talking I was feeling like "Wow, she is so great, I am so glad she is in this group!" How do you feel, though, when people express care or affection or kind words?

> LENORE: I don't believe it. I don't trust it. And I really *want* to believe it! Really, I do.

> GROUP LEADER 2: So, maybe part of your goal would be for you to hear somebody say something like what Sarah just said to you, and to be able to take it in.

Notice that the group leaders do not focus on the interaction between Lenore and Sarah (i.e., the fact that Lenore does not acknowledge Sarah's enthusiastic support), as one might in a psychodynamic interpersonal process group. Rather, they keep the focus on Lenore, highlighting her lack of affect and her constricted response to supportive feedback. This distinction is a rather subtle one, but it is useful to keep in mind when conducting a group based on this model. Group process is addressed not for its own sake, but rather for the sake of clarifying an individual's goal work.

Toward the midpoint of the group therapy, Lenore reveals a secret that she has never disclosed to anyone before. As an adolescent runaway fleeing her abusive home, she was befriended by a pimp who showered her with the care and attention she craved. He then entrapped her into prostitution, subduing her with violent beatings but also with intermittent rewards. She was on the street for 3 years before she managed to escape. In her view, this secret proves that she is irreparably "dirty and disgusting." Group members respond in a caring and accepting manner, again admiring her courage for sharing. The group leaders frame prostitution as a form of exploitation of vulnerable young women, using this moment of psychoeducation to draw attention to the broader social and political context of members' experiences of abuse, in keeping with the TRG's feminist underpinnings. The purpose of such interventions is to shift group members' attributions about such problems from shameful personal flaws that are evidence of "badness" to social problems that affect large numbers of women who have been disempowered by violence and other forms of oppression. Toward the end of her sharing time, group leaders ask Lenore what it has been like to allow the group to know this part of her story. Lenore reports feeling relieved. She does not automatically dismiss the empathetic feedback she has received; but rather, is beginning to take it in.

The goal of "feeling connected" is initially concretized and enacted relationally within the group. The next time she takes a turn to share, Lenore reports that she has been able to expand "feeling connected" in her relationships outside the group as well.

LENORE: So, my goal is for me to feel connected to other people in the group. I don't know if I have anything to talk about. I thought a lot about just being. I seem to have been able to do that all week, which has been really nice. There hasn't been a whole lot of head chatter going on. I am afraid to say that because I feel like I will jinx myself, but it feel likes a little freedom from whatever I have been dragging around for all these years. And I am trying really hard not to be too critical about feeling good. Like, okay, Lenore, you are allowed to feel good. . . . One thing that has happened for me is that I have been seeing this man, and I feel like I have finally allowed for him to care for me, which is really a huge thing for me! It is scary—but not as scary as it was! I can actually possibly see that in my future, whereas I never would have before. It is a whole different kind of relationship. It intrigues me a lot.

GROUP LEADER 1: Can you say a little bit more about how you let him care for you?

LENORE: I think some of it is just letting him in, the trusting. I know that he is really supportive of me and my choices. I think some of it has to do with being here and letting people know me, saying things, and walking away and feeling okay about that. It feels like a weight off at some level. He told me that he saw a change in me. I think Joanne said this a couple weeks ago—that it is very different to talk to a group of people than it is with a therapist.

GROUP LEADER 2: It sounds like taking the risk that you have taken in the group has enabled you to take similar risks in your outside relationships.

LENORE: I feel internally just calmer about things. I have thought a lot about my family and what it was like to grow up and not really have anybody there for me and how that affected me. I think I just feel more at ease with myself and more trusting in the process and not like there is a right or wrong. Some of that judgment that I had on myself just feels less and doesn't feel as harsh, which is a really nice feeling because when I do that I don't judge other people so much.

GROUP LEADER 1: Do you want to open up for feedback?

LENORE: Sure.

JOANNE: I just have to say that everything you say is very exciting to hear. I remember you saying that when you were growing up you never had anyone there for you and that kind of affects you in your relationship with your new partner. I was wondering how it affects you and if you see a change.

LENORE: It definitely affects me, because there was no affection at home when I was growing up. There was hardly any touching at all. So, just regular touching is hard, and allowing that to happen has been nice. Not sex, just touching—and wanting to do that instead of just waiting to get it over with or saying "stop touching me" all the time. I am able to talk to him about it. I tell him everything, which is really nice, really just saying it like it is. Just like—I told him, "I don't want you leaving your clothes at my house," saying things like that. I would not have been able to say that before.

GROUP LEADER 1: It sounds like part of what you are describing are the ways that you have gotten more clarity, both in terms of how you can let him in and also ways in which you can state your need to have some space and privacy. I think it is really wonderful to hear you say how you feel you are changing. What you were able to share with your new friend and how you shared in the group 2 weeks ago sound very much related.

ANDREA: I think I remember you saying "I want to know myself," and now you are finding out new things about yourself: you can communicate, you can be touched, and be happy. How does that make you feel?

LENORE: There is a piece of myself that has been just dormant that feels like it is finally coming alive. It is not about that I have a man now. That is not what it is, it is just about me.

In the final session, Lenore sums up her achievements in the group. She has accomplished her goal of "feeling connected"—first, by revealing to the group a closely guarded secret from her past life, and second, through a complex process of internalizing the viewpoint of the other group members. Because she is able to feel compassion and affection for the other group members, she is now also able to imagine herself in the eyes of another person who regards her with affection and compassion. As she does so, she experiences relief from her chronic feeling of intense shame, her sense of being "dirty and disgusting." This transformation in a survivor's sense of self-in-relation is a major achievement of the second stage of recovery.

"So, what did I come here to achieve? I was really scared to start this group because I knew I was ready to unearth some things. So, I had a lot of trepidation about what that was going to mean. I also really wanted to start feeling more connected to people and feel more in touch with myself and feel more grounded. I really needed to let people in a little bit more, and I feel like I have achieved that. So, I feel really good about that. The biggest things for me are the benefits of not keeping a secret and being able to talk about things that I thought that if I ever talked about them I would melt and disappear into the ground or people would go scurrying from the room like rats. And I found that didn't happen, both for me and for other people. I can almost step outside of myself now and look at the circumstances, because I know how I would respond if someone told me my story. I would feel really sad for that person—so I hope I can keep that perspective. I feel like I am viewing myself kinder and not as judgmental."

As she feels less ashamed, Lenore is also able to let go of her defensive, judgmental attitude toward others. She has become more aware of the ways that she has kept others at a distance, and as she finds new ways to allow them to know her better, she feels more "connected." This is an illustration of the power of experiencing safe attachment in the TRG therapy and in transforming members' expectations about interpersonal relationships.

LENORE: The other really big thing is I feel like I am less judgmental and critical of myself, and I have compassion toward myself and toward others. I realized how judgmental I really am of both myself and other people. That is what I sort of discovered: I was judging other people because I was so hard on myself, and I feel like that has really changed and something switched for me. The biggest thing is that I definitely feel more connected to people everywhere.

GROUP LEADER 1: Do you feel ready to hear other people's reflections on your process?

SARAH: First I want to thank you for the feelings you have shared in this group. I want you to believe me when I tell you that this is sincerely from a caring and loving place in my heart that I hope the fact that you have revealed the secret that has burdened you so long and that you have acknowledged the pain and suffering you have had around those circumstances results in a freedom from fear and anxiety in both your body and your mind and also from the fear of being unknowable and unknown, unlovable and unloved. I hope you continue to resist judging yourself so harshly and that your mind and body will be free of anxiety and self-doubt. I hope you can instead continue to feel supported by the validation from the members of this group, that you are not alone and that you can hold on to the care and kindness that you have experienced and received here. And I hope that this experience will be part of a lasting, firm foundation of a better relationship with other people who care deeply about you. And finally, it is my hope that you can acknowledge that you deserve to be happy, that you deserve to be loved and cared for with tenderness and appreciation for the wonderful person that you are.

ANDREA: I basically agree with everything Sarah said, but I think you also said something about compassion and being compassionate to yourself, and I think that is a key word for me to give you as a gift, which I think you really have given yourself, to—no matter what—be compassionate to yourself.

JOANNE: You said that you came here to be more connected, to make relationships in here, and then in your outside life. It has been exciting to watch your progress. You are kind of like a role model, and you really did what you came here to do! When you first came here, you were a lot more closed, and, to be honest, I found you a little intimidating. You seemed really stressed and tense and harsh, and now you are so much more relaxed, and it is just really different. So, I hope that the love that is entering into your life will just expand and make it so that you will be able to be this way with whomever you choose. I feel very hopeful that it will happen, because just look at all you have accomplished in the last 4 months!

GROUP LEADER 1: Do you experience a difference in being in your body? Because a number of people have referenced *that*. Can you take in what people are saying?

LENORE: That is the difference—I can take it in.

COMMON CHALLENGES

Not every case will progress in such a straightforward fashion. Group members' goal work can be derailed in any number of ways. Here we address some of the problems that are most commonly encountered during this phase of TRG therapy.

A Member Is Unable to Settle on a Goal

Although most members are able to identify their goal and refine it sufficiently by this stage, sometimes one or more members are still struggling to decide on a goal or to make it specific and concrete enough to be achievable within the time limits of the therapy. If a group member is still floundering in terms of goal definition while other group members are progressing, it can lead to considerable distress during the sessions and a sense of incompletion at the end.

At this point, it may be helpful to take time to explore what makes the process of formulating a goal so difficult. For example, one member indicated that her difficulty in selecting a goal reflected her broader difficulty in knowing her thoughts, feelings, and preferences. Group leaders and members invited her to reflect on the aspects of her history that may have contributed to this broader difficulty and how it affects her current life. This discussion led to her identifying a goal of being attentive to her thoughts, feelings, and preferences during the group sessions and sharing her observations with the group. On occasion, a member will struggle with a lack of confidence in her ability to remain focused or to achieve success. At such times, normalization of these negative expectations resulting from shame and other sequelae of interpersonal abuse or neglect coupled with empathetic encouragement can help her to feel more able to progress.

If this in-group process is not successful, it may be necessary for the group leaders to meet with a member for a session outside of group to help her formulate her goal. In such instances, it is always important that the rest of group be aware that such a meeting is taking place. Ideally, the plan for an extra meeting should be devised during the group's session. Alternatively, if the group member is in individual therapy, the group leaders might suggest that the member use this therapy to work on her goal, and they might offer to confer with her individual therapist.

A Goal Appears Unreachable as Originally Defined

As the goal work phase progresses, it sometimes becomes apparent that a member's goal is too ambitious, given the pace of work and the duration of the therapy. As an example, a member who has identified a goal of disclosing to her whole family her history of incest may realize that she is not ready for the range of potential reactions to such a disclosure. Since the experience of success and mastery is central to the curative process of the group, it is important to help the member redefine her goal so that it is achievable. This redefinition is also important in helping the client understand the importance of paying attention to pacing and timing during this stage of recovery. In this case, the member may decide that she instead will disclose only to the therapy group or in addition perhaps to one friend or family member whom she anticipates will be supportive. Her work in the group can thus be framed as an important step toward a larger goal of more extensive disclosure.

A Member Has Difficulty in Remaining Focused on Her Goal

As cohesion increases, members often long for general mutual support and expanded sharing. Real-life difficulties in the present unrelated to members' specific goals may compete for their attention and press to be shared with the group. Members may have difficulty in containing some of their associations to the experiences shared by others, although these may not be related to the goal work that they have defined for themselves. Reminding members to begin their sharing turn by restating their goal can be helpful in addressing these difficulties. Co-leaders need to be prepared to interrupt and redirect members by inquiring how what is being shared is related to the member's goal. The group leaders should validate the importance of these competing concerns and encourage the member to seek support through individual therapy or other resources. If a member repeatedly strays from her goal, it may be necessary to reevaluate the relevance of the particular goal she has chosen in light of the client's current life circumstances, which may have significantly changed over the course of the therapy.

A Member Becomes Overwhelmed by Trauma Memories

It is important that the group leaders have sufficient experience in treating complexly traumatized clients so as to be able to distinguish between a member who is experiencing painful affect as she works through memories of the trauma and one who is flooded or overwhelmed. Some indicators that a client is becoming flooded include the experience of flashbacks and intense reliving experiences in group sessions, manifesting in notable difficulties in distinguishing past from present. A client who is overwhelmed may also display indications of dissociation, such as an inability to make eye contact or appearing "spaced out" or "shut down," difficulty in recalling parts of a session, losing the ability to use words to describe her experiences, a marked shift in appearance, and expressing a feeling of disconnection from herself and other members. A member who is in a highly activated or dissociated affective state is unable to benefit from telling the trauma narrative in a relational context because her information-processing capacities are compromised. In the event that a group member becomes too affectively overwhelmed while sharing her trauma narrative, the group leaders can offer suggestions for grounding (e.g., taking a few deep breaths, putting feet on the floor, looking around the room) and assist the member in moving into a more "cognitive" position from which she can reflect upon her reaction. This approach is usually sufficiently containing; however, if group leaders are still concerned about the member by the end of the session, they should check in with her between sessions and follow up with her individual therapist as needed. It is important that the group be aware that the co-leaders are attending to the distressed member so that they do not leave the session worrying about her.

The Group Tries to "Rescue" Members from Painful Affect

Connecting with affect is an important part of processing and integrating traumatic experiences; however, it may feel frightening for many group members. Members will sometimes try to "rescue" someone who is crying or otherwise expressing emotional pain by intervening quickly to reassure her, expressing anger toward the perpetrator, asking a contextual question, or offering a practical solution. In such instances, the group leaders should verbally acknowledge the helpful intention of such interventions as well as how hard it is to experience the feelings of sadness, anger, and helplessness sometimes evoked within the group. They should also mention that such interventions can serve to distract the member from processing important emotions related to the trauma. This observation usually helps to contain the group and build its affect tolerance.

Difficulties with Time Keeping

Although time-keeping problems may arise at any point in the group, they may be hardest to manage when members start to talk in more depth about their traumatic experiences and related affect. It is hard to interrupt a member who is experiencing intense affect or to cut short empathetic feedback. However, one must remember that the structure of the group conveys a sense of safety and predictability as members do this demanding Stage 2 work, and that the intention is to provide members with an experience of mutuality. As such, group leaders are responsible for ensuring that each session begins and ends on time, that the group time is shared equally among members, and that there is adequate time for feedback. It may be helpful for the group leaders to agree prior to each session who will be responsible for the time keeping. It is important that a group leader intervene approximately halfway though a member's sharing time to ask whether she is ready for feedback if she does not get to this point by herself. It is also helpful to remind the whole group when only 5 minutes remain of a member's turn, in order to facilitate the transition to the next speaker. Group leaders should discuss any repeated difficulties with time-keeping issues with their supervisor.

A Member Avoids Taking Her Turn in Sharing

As far as possible, group leaders should hold members to the expectation that they will take time to share their goal work with the group on a regular rotating basis. It happens occasionally that members request to "pass" in a particular session or offer their time to another member who appears to be having difficulty or needing more support. There are circumstances in which this type of change may be appropriate. Some exchanges are likely to happen during the course of therapy, and it is important for the group to remain flexible in this regard. For example, a group member disclosed during the check-in that an abusive ex-boyfriend had begun calling and threatening her during the week, causing her great distress. Another member offered her the use of her time during the session to process her reactions. The offer was gratefully accepted, and the group agreed that trading turns would be acceptable in this situation.

We do not recommend frequent time trading, however, nor do we advise that a member attend more than two consecutive sessions without claiming sharing time. Repeated efforts to forgo taking a turn may reflect avoidance of trauma-related material or the intimacy of the group or other relational difficulties that may have some relevance to the member's goal.

A Group Member's Continued Participation Is Questioned

Questions occasionally arise about whether a member's continued participation would be contraindicated for her and/or for the group, although thorough screening minimizes the frequency of this problem. Examples may include a member who becomes extremely symptomatic, raising concerns about her safety or possible hospitalization, or a member who is interpersonally overly hostile or excessively disruptive. In such instances, the first course of action is to consult with the member's individual therapist, followed by a meeting of both co-leaders with the member. Through these contacts, the co-leaders can explore whether anything can be done to contain the member and enable her to continue her group work. For example, if the member is engaging in outside activities that are particularly stressful or triggering, could she postpone those activities until the TRG therapy has ended? Alternatively, if the member is feeling angry and dealing with anger is relevant to her goal, could she take some time to express her feelings with some prior coaching from her individual therapist in the most appropriate way to do so? In our experience, it is usually possible to salvage a member's participation in such a way that she is still able to feel that she did some important work within the group. However, it is conceivable that situations will arise where this is not possible and, if this is the case, the client should leave the group. In such an instance, the co-leaders should take ample time during the next group session to process members' reactions fully.

Out-of-Group Contacts

Actively discouraging out-of-group contacts among members is an important position to uphold for the entire course of TRG therapy, to provide group members with needed safety and structure. During the goal-work stage of the therapy, members may long for and subtly attempt to increase their contacts with other members before and after the group sessions. This type of information may come to the group leaders' attention through a member who is feeling left out or through their own direct observation of interactions in the waiting room or parking lot. Group leaders should address this breach of the group guidelines at the first indication that it is occurring, reminding members of the reasons for this rule. It may be helpful to add that, although increased contacts may feel goal-oriented or particularly supportive during a period of difficulty, their overall effect is detrimental to the group process and to individuals' opportunities to maximize the insights gained during group sessions as a whole. The co-leaders should remind members that they will have the option of sharing their contact information with other members when the therapy ends. All group members should also be apprised of any significant out-of-group contacts with the co-leaders—for example, if co-leaders have to meet with someone outside of the group to discuss an obstacle to her full participation.

CONCLUSION

The middle phase of TRG therapy is characterized by great emotional intensity as members become immersed in the trauma-focused work of the second stage of recovery and as they pursue the goals they selected for themselves during the introductory phase. The art of group leadership during this phase is to keep a clear focus on each group member's goal, even as she shares painful memories of the past, and to foster affective exchanges that deepen mutual understanding and a sense of connection to others. By planning an action in the present and then executing on that plan, each group member seeks to overcome the feeling of powerlessness often engendered by trauma. Most commonly group members find that a goal that initially seemed impossible to achieve in isolation becomes increasingly attainable with the support of their TRG peers, resulting in growing feelings of mastery and empowerment.

CHAPTER 6

The Concluding Phase

The third and final phase of the TRG involves concluding therapy. At the end of the 12th or start of the 13th session, group co-leaders should remind members that they will each have only one more turn to complete their goal or review their completed goal work and receive feedback before the group transitions into a closing exercise that will take place over the last two sessions. Appendix H (Time-Taking Tracking Tool) should be helpful in clarifying the timing of this announcement. In the TRG model, the concluding phase is as much about ending one's treatment with a sense of mastery as it is about saying good-bye.

For some members, the impending end-of-group treatment provides a special impetus for accomplishing their goals. For example, one member who had set a goal of being able to talk about her childhood rape without dissociating avoided doing so until this final phase of the therapy by talking instead about the ways in which it had affected her life. The reminder that the group would soon be ending prompted the client to "pluck up the courage" to relate these events to the group in a thoroughly connected way. Another member sent a letter of confrontation that she had originally thought she could write only to herself (as an exercise in expressing her sense of reality). She had discovered during the TRG therapy that she had far more emotional supports in her life than she had realized, and so she decided that in the event the letter received a negative response, she nonetheless would be able to handle the consequences because both the letter's writing and its sending were really "just for her."

Members who have already accomplished their goals may use these later sessions to reflect on their experience of having done so successfully—and the impact of that realization on their lives. For example, a member who had achieved her goal of revealing to her partner portions of her trauma history that she had previously kept secret—and experiencing his acceptance and appreciation of her—used the remaining sessions to reflect on the impact of her heightened self-disclosure on her daily relationship with him. This process helped amplify her awareness that the disclosure had actually created a more open and trusting relationship between the two of them.

For certain members, the imminent approach of the group's ending date may lead to the realization that their original goal will not be fully accomplished. In that case, their work during the remaining sessions should be to identify worthwhile steps that have been taken in the right direction so that they still end the treatment with a sense of mastery. Thus, group leaders will need to be active in assisting any such member in identifying an important action step that she took or some important understanding that she gained over the course of the therapy. Group leaders should come well prepared to the last goal work session in case one or more participants is at a loss in terms of recognizing her accomplishments. For example, one member had identified a goal of developing self-empathy and had struggled to find a clear-cut way to assess whether she had succeeded in doing so. She was reminded by other members that she had shown enormous empathy in working with her peers in the group. One of the co-leaders asked her if she was aware of any ways she had been able to experience these feelings toward herself. She offered the description below, and the other group leader suggested that she have someone write it down so that she would have tangible evidence of having accomplished something worthwhile in the TRG.

> "I guess when you put it that way, it's probably true. I never blamed anyone else in the group for what had happened to them; so, maybe I can start to give myself a break instead of thinking it was all my fault. And because I can be myself here, I've gotten more relaxed with people at work, where I used to feel that if they knew me they'd find out my secret. But when I'm with people in the group, they just seem like regular women to me, their secrets aren't visible to the world, and so mine probably aren't either. And I think of the women in this group as so courageous in surviving what had happened and then coming to therapy to work on it; so, maybe some of that courage is in me too."

PREPARING FOR CONCLUSION OF THE TRG

In preparing for the conclusion sessions, the group leaders should claim some time to (1) speak about the concluding exercise and (2) discuss the issue of out-of-group contacts. In Session 14 (the third-to-last session), the group leaders present and explain the concluding exercise that will structure the final two sessions. While a shorter-term group (with 10 or 12 sessions) can conceivably conduct this termination process in one session, two sessions seem to be optimal for members to reflect on their progress and receive feedback from others. The question of out-of-group contacts is usually addressed at the beginning or end of Session 15 so that members have an opportunity to consider their preferences before the final therapy session ends.

Introducing the Concluding Exercise

At the end of the 14th session, members are given a "homework" assignment and provided with psychoeducation about the closing agenda for the group. They are told that the last two sessions follow a somewhat different format, and they are each asked to consider the following questions in relation to *themselves and every other member* of the group:

"What was my goal?"
"What did I accomplish in relation to my original goal?"
"What might be a possible next step I will take as a result of being in this group?"
"What imaginary gift will I give to myself related to my work in this group?"

To aid memory, it may be helpful to write the questions on a poster board or to list them on a handout that is distributed to group members (see the sample provided in Appendix I). Similarly, members may want to write down their feedback if this helps to organize their thinking. Whether their thoughts are put into written form or not, co-leaders should make it clear that members are expected to spend time thinking hard about their own and others' work in the group. They should also ask group members to prepare to share general feedback about the whole TRG experience, and let the group know that the leaders will prepare feedback for each group member.

At this time, members sometimes raise the question of *gift giving* at the close of the therapy. The "imaginary gift" concept was developed in response to this issue, because even small symbolic gifts can sometimes give rise to competitive or guilty feelings. Co-leaders should encourage members to think of their words—feedback and support—as the best and most valuable gift to one another. Imaginary gifts (e.g., an imaginary loudspeaker given to a member who struggles with self-assertion, or an emotional raincoat for dealing with upsetting interactions with family members) can be an effective way to express farewell wishes for some group members.

Discussing Out-of-Group Contacts

Another important issue that should be addressed in the second- or third-to-last session is the question of out-of-group contacts. As the end of the group therapy approaches, some members express a desire to sustain the relationships that they have developed over the course of the treatment. During the 15th session, the leaders should raise the topic of pursuing out-of-group contacts for those who wish to stay connected. It is helpful for co-leaders to acknowledge and validate this desire while at the same time providing members with some psychoeducational points to consider as they think about whether to pursue contacts with their peers after the group has ended. The leaders should remind members that the decision about whether or not to pursue out-of-group contacts is very personal and may vary from one member to the next. Some may wish to continue the relationships that evolved over the course of the therapy, whereas others may prefer to preserve the memory of the connections that they experienced without taking them any further. Some may feel wary about continuing the relationships without the presence and guidance of the co-leaders. The importance of respecting individual decisions should be emphasized. For those who choose not to extend their peer relationships and do so apologetically, group leaders should support their boundary setting and urge other members to do likewise. They should emphasize that this choice should not be interpreted as a signal that the relationships were not important but rather may be a different way of holding on to the connections.

Leaders should be prepared to intervene if there is any shaming, blaming, or teasing behavior during this discussion. They should also remind group members that, although they may continue to have supportive relationships with one another after the group has ended, it will no longer be therapy, and therefore the connections are likely to feel quite different. Sharing intimate personal information with intense feelings may no longer be appropriate; however, members may want to try out a more lighthearted way of socializing with one another. Options should be discussed for those who might change their mind about participating later in continued contact. A simple "I no longer wish to have contact should suffice.

Members should also be informed that another important implication of posttreatment out-of-group contacts is that they may be denied the option of participating in a future round of the TRG, as including two or more members with outside relationships would create in-group and out-group dynamics that would not work well in this goal-focused model.

CONCLUDING SESSIONS

The last two sessions begin and end in the usual way, with the opening and closing rounds. The leaders should claim about 10 minutes in the second-to-last session to speak about out-of-group contacts, as discussed above. The remaining time is divided among half the members, and each member begins her turn by sharing her reflections on her own progress with reference to the earlier cited questions (which should be repeated at the outset by group leaders). Once the first person finishes her assessment (taking about one-third of her allotted time), feedback should be invited from group members based on their reflections. Although note taking during sessions is discouraged at other times, during the concluding session group members may want to have the feedback that they receive from others recorded for future reference. It is helpful to have someone else in the group record it for them so that they can remain focused on receiving the feedback, letting themselves both hear it and experience the feelings that arise in this process. Some members may need help from the leaders or peers to really take in all the positive feedback, and occasional interjections like "Are you taking it in?" and "Do you need us to slow down?" can be helpful. The person recording the feedback should alternate for each member who is sharing, as this may otherwise result in that person's participating less in the group. This concluding exercise should include opportunities for the member to respond to the feedback, time allowing. It is ideal for each member to receive feedback from most if not all other members of the group, although members should be encouraged to add new feedback, if possible, rather than repeat what has already been said.

It is usually best for group leaders to give their feedback last, as it often happens that much of their feedback has already been articulated meaningfully by group members. However, it is crucially important that the group leaders remain active both in encouraging all members to provide their feedback and address questions, and in managing the time carefully so that each member can receive feedback from a number of different people. It is important that the co-leaders give prior thought to and discuss with each other the feedback they intend to provide to each member. Each co-leader takes a primary role in providing feedback to half of the members of the group, making it clear that she is speaking on behalf of both therapists and delivering feedback that they prepare together. She should add any important observations that have been left out (referring to a specific memory about the member's work whenever possible). This occasion is one of the times in the treatment when co-leaders can fully appreciate the advantage of keeping detailed weekly notes. It is highly validating to be able to speak about a member's goal-work progress in very concrete and specific terms.

Case Example: Angela

Angela was sexually abused by her father, a high-powered and highly esteemed academic in the field of anthropology. During the TRG therapy she wrote him a letter in which she confronted him with her memories of the abuse he had perpetrated. He replied with a letter written on stationery from his Ivy League institution. It was a reflection on the role of memory in various tribal groups and the need for people to create "narrative myths" to explain the unhappiness or unfortunate circumstances in their lives. He concluded that he was so sorry that Angela had had to resort to this practice to explain her bad marriage. She shared his letter with the group, and the rest of her work included figuring out her next step in relation to him. Instead of entering into an argument with him, she decided that his denial meant he could not spend time with her children unsupervised. If he chose to get treatment, she would rely on his therapist to decide if and when this course of action might change.

As part of her concluding session, the group leaders were able to give her a detailed account of the session in which she brought in his letter and shared it with the group. They reminded her that she at first had felt shattered and then scared that he might be correct. Although she had expressed little hope about his confirming her memories, she had yearned for validation. When the group was unimpressed by his academic jargon, offering feedback such as "Nice try, buddy" and "Imagine, he's a fancy professor, and he managed to say the same thing as my father, the plumber!," she gradually regained her confidence and her self-doubt disappeared. The leaders told her that exposure to the validation of others seemed to be a good remedy for her to employ when he tried to undermine her again, as he inevitably would.

Sometimes goal work is unfinished, and leaders need to reframe the work so that the member leaves with a sense of mastery. This reframing process involves reviewing the member's progress for an accomplished piece of work regarding her goal so that each participant will feel a sense of mastery, which is vitally important to the overall purpose of the group. This reframing is accomplished much more easily if the co-leaders have helped the member imagine breaking her goal down into manageable steps earlier during the therapy (as described in Chapter 5) than if they have to try to do this downsizing retrospectively.

Case Example: Priscilla

Priscilla had come to the group with the goal of confronting her elderly father with the details of the abuse she had suffered at his hands and the impact it had had on her life. Although she believed that this could harm him because of his age, she felt it was important to confront him while she still had the opportunity. She began preparing for the event in group sessions, deciding what to say and how to take care of herself. During the course of her therapy, he developed a terminal illness. After a lot of thought, Priscilla decided to abandon the plan because she believed that her family's condemnation of her for "hurting such a sick man" would be more difficult for her to bear than any psychological gain from speaking her truth to him directly. Leaders and group members saw this as a wise decision and pointed out that she'd accomplished a lot by determining how best to move forward with her family under the new circumstances. One co-leader reminded her that she had in fact disclosed her history to an aunt while preparing to confront her father directly. Even though she had anticipated that this aunt would be supportive, she had not known for certain until she made the disclosure. That she had taken this important step successfully was key to the mastery of her goal. The group leaders highlighted this event, which had occurred midway through therapy, and stated that they believed her success indicated that Priscilla had the tools she needed to disclose to or confront family members whenever the time was right for her.

"Next Steps"

The "next steps" recommended by co-leaders may be general or specific and often include a framing psychoeducational explanation specific to each client. The advice may involve recommendations about joining other groups that may be beneficial to the client in continuing her work (e.g., an interpersonal process group, another trauma-related group) or suggestions about areas that should be explored further in individual therapy. For some clients, this feedback may involve nonclinical recommendations, such as taking on volunteer work or becoming involved in a social group. It is usually recommended that even clients who may benefit from participating in another group first take some time to process their accomplishments in the present group and their implications. Case examples of feedback regarding these different types of recommended next steps follow.

Penny: Further Work in Individual Therapy as a Next Step

Penny's goal in the group had been to verify further her memories of a babysitter's abuse of both herself and her sister by approaching old neighbors to see whether any of them remembered him or had concerns about her parents hiring him. She was able to find two people who had known him and her family. They recalled that he had been asked to leave the Boy Scouts because of his behavior with his young charges and said they had wondered why her parents kept using him as a babysitter when this news became known in the neighborhood. In reflecting on her progress and next steps, Penny expressed a desire to disclose her memories (and this information that she had recently obtained) to her sister. Group members and leaders supported her moving in this direction but encouraged her to work further in individual therapy to prepare for this disclosure. Penny felt that she risked her sister's denial—which would be harmful to her—or bringing on an emotional breakdown on her sister's part, for which she would then feel responsible. Further exploration of what these consequences might entail for her own recovery was thus indicated before taking any action.

Claudia: Another Therapy Group as a Next Step

As she concluded the TRG therapy and reflected on her work, Claudia wondered about whether she had become too much the caretaker in her relationship with her partner. In working on a goal related to increasing her self-care, Claudia became more aware of the impact of her role as the eldest daughter in a large family with a mentally ill mother and alcoholic and abusive stepfather. Aided by feedback from other members, she also recognized the caretaking role she often assumed in the group, putting her needs aside in favor of others. As a next step, the group leaders encouraged Claudia to look for an ongoing interpersonal psychotherapy group where she could further explore this role and experiment with different ways of relating to others. In Claudia's case, she was advised that it could be a women's group or a mixed-gender group. We believe that developing relationship skills and building capacity for intimacy is work that can be done in either kind of group, depending on the needs and preferences of the particular client. We have found that for such a referral to be helpful at least one of the co-leaders of the group receiving the referral should be experienced in trauma work and knowledgeable about the impact of previous trauma on present-day relationships.

Rebecca: A Nonclinical Next Step

Rebecca was successful in her job as a clinical social worker. When her daughter turned 4, the age at which Rebecca had been molested, she began to have disturbing flashbacks and nightmares. She was often tired, and her nerves were constantly triggered by her clients. She had always known about the abuse and had worked on it in individual therapy, but she had not anticipated that sensing her daughter's vulnerability would cause old symptoms to return, as she was in a good marriage and felt good about her parenting skills. She decided to leave her job, and when she began the TRG she felt as though she had given into the perpetrator by allowing him to render her a failure professionally. Her goal for the TRG was to reappraise this action as one she had taken in the interest of self-care and as a wise choice she had made on behalf of herself and her family. She accomplished her goal, and as a next step the co-leaders suggested that she consider engaging in volunteer work, perhaps at her daughter's school, where many of her skills would be utilized and she could feel appreciated and competent without the demands of a full-time job. She left feeling quite excited about this prospect.

Concluding Exercise: An Illustrative Transcript

In the following abbreviated transcript of an excerpt from a concluding session of the TRG, Olivia reflects on her progress and receives feedback from group members and co-leaders. Olivia's goal in the therapy was to be able to talk about her experience of childhood sexual abuse by her father with sense of connection to and awareness of her affective responses.

OLIVIA: I always thought it would kill me if I told my story with my real feelings attached to it. I knew what happened and could say it all in detail, and I knew what I felt—devastated, ashamed, dirty, guilty. I wanted the contact; I was so starved for attention, and I would initiate it a lot of the time. I was sick to my stomach at the thought of how much I feared him and how much I loved him. My mother was really crazy and verbally assaultive and neglectful and just plain mean. So, these feelings would wash over me at any time of the day or night but not really associated with any memories or anything. Just shame and guilt, feeling dirty, all the time. Except when I'd tell about it and laugh, like it was a weird story about somebody else. So, when you guys suggested this goal, I was really mad because all I wanted was to be here and relax; it's nice to be with other people who've experienced similar things. I know you meant well, but it took me a while to realize that you really believed I could tell my story and have my feelings at the same time and that the people in the group would witness my reality and that would really help me. So, I decided to try it and see how it went, knowing I could always stop and there would be people to help me if I really flipped out. And it did help! I sobbed and sobbed and was angry at the right times; I never thought I could tell about how when I got married he told me that I always asked for it, and how he'd taught me about healthy sexuality and my husband would appreciate him for it. I felt so much relief when the group didn't turn from me in disgust but expressed total sympathy and thought he should rot in hell—and I knew they were right! So, I can see a different future for myself, and I am so grateful to all the women in this group and the therapists. Knowing that I can accomplish goals means that the next steps for me will be working on my marriage. He's been so there for me, but I constantly push him away for fear he's like my father underneath, because on the surface my father was a great guy too. I just want to hang out with my husband and notice what I feel when I'm with him, now that I can trust myself to put words to my feelings, should I need to. We might need help in couples counseling; we might not. I'd like to see what happens. A gift I could give myself is a cloud that rains words and a lion that roars words, so when I'm sad the cloud will rain with my sad words, and when I'm angry the lion will roar my angry words.

TRISH: I remember when you started sobbing as you told your story, and it seemed like you might not stop and that is what I've always been afraid of, myself . . . but you did stop and you said you felt so relieved and that was so powerful for me to witness. . . . I thank you so much. I'm glad you'll focus on your marriage. I wish for you a hammock that represents the group, and when you need us you get in the hammock and we surround you with support.

WANDA: You go, girl! You certainly did your goal! I like you so much better with your feelings connected. You used to seem pretty numb sometimes. I'm happy you have a good man in your life, and my gift to you is a beautiful long beach where the two of you can walk hand in hand. And if that doesn't work, I have a good marriage counselor for you!

ZOEY: We were paired in the exercise that first day; so, I always felt a special attachment to you and sort of like I wanted to look out for you. You seemed scared a lot, but you could never say what you were scared of until you did your goal work in the group. It's so great to feel you have so much strength on your own! My imaginary gift to you is a doll that looks like you, and when you pull a string it says, "I know what I feel, I know what I feel!" (*Everyone laughs.*)

LUCY: From the beginning, even before you could name your feelings, I totally got that you felt so much shame because you sought your father out sometimes. And I was so mad because you were a little girl and you wanted affection, and I know it can feel like affection. And then there's the physical pleasure aspect, and as you grew older your body does respond whether you want it to or not—but that has nothing to do with wanting it. It's like your body has betrayed you—but that's not it; it's *your father* who betrayed you! And you see how worked up I get so I didn't say this to you, but I'm telling you now because you didn't deserve any of it! You are a great person, and I gift you a mirror that always shows you how spectacular you are!

MARTHA: It's all been said, so I won't repeat it. My gift to you is one of the DVDs that teach kids about their feelings and why feelings are good and okay, so you can always know that.

CO-LEADER 1: I just want to add that my experience of watching you come to trust the group and us enough to hold you as you did your goal work was a gift. Your struggle and determination were evident even when you doubted whether this process would be helpful. It took a leap of faith on your part, and I so appreciate the faith you put in us.

CO-LEADER 2: Our joint gift to you is a private studio to do the art work that is now spread over your dining room table. It has many windows with abundant light streaming in, and you have all the supplies you need and time to devote to your art.

OLIVIA: (*tearfully*) Thank you, all of you. I couldn't have done this alone.

ENDING THE FINAL SESSION

Some 10–15 minutes should be reserved at the end of the final session for the group leaders to get feedback from members regarding their general experience of participating in this particular group. This feedback may include comments about aspects of the group and its leadership that were particularly helpful as well as sources of frustration or disappointment. The group co-leaders should also use this time to express some well-considered thoughts about their experience of facilitating this group. The final group session ends with the co-leaders exiting the room first, leaving members to exchange contact information with one another if they so desire.

CONCLUDING CONTACTS WITH INDIVIDUAL/PRIMARY THERAPISTS

Prior to the final session, the group leaders should contact each member's individual therapist to let him or her know that the group is ending and share their observations about the member's work as well as recommendations for next steps. If participating in another group is one of the recommendations, group leaders should either make the appropriate referral or provide the individual therapist with the information needed to do so.

CONCLUSION

Group members usually experience the termination process as a gift in itself. Each person is the center of attention for a while, and the process is completely designed to celebrate each one's accomplishments within the group. Each person also gets valuable information about her worth in the eyes of other group members and their recognition for the role she played in their own healing. The concluding self-assessment exercise gives members a tangible means of focusing on what they were able to achieve as opposed to the negative self-evaluation that is so common among survivors. Having had the experience of identifying a goal and refining it so that it is manageable and achievable (as described in Chapter 4) as well as processing trauma memories related to this goal in a safe, gradually paced, and relationally attuned way (as illustrated in Chapter 5), members end the treatment with a sense of mastery and confidence in their ability to handle other tasks of recovery. They move forward with a feeling of empowerment—a sense that their choices and actions can effect real change in their lives—and the experience of having been worthy and contributing members of a much valued community. These achievements are emblematic of the feminist influence on the TRG and the treatment's ultimate aim of helping victims become active survivors.

CHAPTER 7

Supervision

In Chapter 2, we provided a rationale for why we consider supervision or consultation a key element in successfully implementing the TRG. Apart from the benefits of supervision in clinical work in general and in group therapy and trauma treatment in particular, the supervisor in this instance helps to ensure that the co-leaders implement the key features of the TRG treatment model effectively. The supervisor maintains the goal focus of the group, assisting co-leaders in tracking the progress of individual members and identifying interventions that might be helpful in defining, refining, and preparing members to act upon their goals. The supervisor also ensures that the group maintains its trauma focus; that the present-oriented goals selected by clients are related to experiences of past trauma; and that their pursuit involves the processing of trauma memories. He or she provides a venue for group leaders to reflect on the emotional impact of hearing members' stories and to identify ways to take better care of themselves and each other. The supervisor pays attention to the overall trajectory of the group and the tasks that need to be accomplished in each phase from preparation and screening through termination. He or she also supports group leaders in maintaining the structure of time sharing and fulfilling their responsibilities with regard to time management within sessions. The supervisor helps co-leaders to maximize the supportive process and to understand group dynamics and use them when appropriate to further members' goal work. Finally, supervision provides a forum in which co-leadership dynamics can be discussed, evaluated, and addressed to increase the comfort of group leaders and thus their effectiveness within the group.

SUPERVISOR CHARACTERISTICS AND REQUIREMENTS

The TRG should ideally be supervised by a clinician who has had prior experience using this group model. If this is not possible, the supervisor should have prior experience in supervising trauma treatment and conducting and supervising other groups for trauma survivors. He or she should thus have some familiarity with the challenges and benefits of group treatment with this population. Prior to agreeing to supervise the group, the supervisor should have thoroughly familiarized him- or herself with the treatment guide and should understand and be able to explain the six key components of the treatment model. In addition, he or she should have a clear understanding of what constitutes an appropriate goal and be able to convey this information clearly. The TRG may be quite different from other groups with which clinicians may be more familiar (such as psychoeducational, support, or process groups), and aspects of the treatment model can initially seem counterintuitive. Supervisees often find it helpful for the supervisor to be very clear and direct about the ways in which this group differs from other models (see Chapters 1 and 2). It is important that the supervisor like and have confidence in the model and be able to communicate this sense of confidence to the co-leaders.

The recommended knowledge foundations and characteristics of the co-leaders described in Chapter 2 are also required of group supervisors. Additionally, the supervisor should have an understanding of the dynamics and challenges involved in co-leadership (for a review, see Delucia-Waack & Fauth, 2004). As far as possible, the supervisor should not have a dual relationship with one co-leader (e.g., he or she should not be a close colleague or that person's supervisor in another context). If this arrangement proves unavoidable, the relationship should be openly acknowledged, and the supervisor should be especially attentive to how this relationship might affect the dynamics of his or her supervisory function.

It is advisable that any first-time supervisor of a TRG observe as many sessions as possible. Although this arrangement might seem potentially disruptive to the group, we have found that, when properly prepared in advance, members are usually quite receptive to a visit from the supervisor and can feel even more secure that their co-leaders are getting the support that they need. We recommend that co-leaders prepare potential group members for a supervisor's visit during the screening phase and initial session by saying something like the following:

> "This group will be supervised by a therapist experienced in group trauma treatment so that the leaders will have someone to whom they can bring any questions or concerns, as well as to share successes. In every group we learn more about how to be helpful to our group members, and this learning is even greater when we are able to discuss our observations with a supervisor. Our supervisor will visit the group from time to time and observe us as we work with you. This will help [him or her] to give us guidance. [He or she] will not be coming here to evaluate your progress but rather to provide us with feedback on how we can be most helpful to the group."

When a supervisor visits a session, he or she is introduced and then sits quietly and unobtrusively outside of the group members' circle, observing the session while taking notes. At the end of the session, he or she may make brief comments appreciating/validating/supporting members' work and appreciating their willingness to have him or her attend the session. It is our experience that the members feel validated by knowing that so much time and attention are being given to their recovery, and they easily adapt to the supervisor's presence in the room. The co-leaders may feel slightly more uncomfortable and be concerned about being judged. It is important for the supervisor to develop a collaborative working relationship with the co-leaders. In supplying them with useful feedback, the supervisor should say what he or she appreciated in the various interventions of each leader as well as suggested options for more effective leadership. This feedback should be as substantive and behaviorally oriented as possible. For example, instead of saying "I liked your warmth and caring stance toward Cathy," the supervisor might say, "I liked that when Cathy came in and seemed unsure about where to sit because her seat from last week was taken, you said her name, smiled, and pointed to a seat that was unoccupied." When advising a different intervention than the one the supervisor employed, instead of saying "You should have been more direct with Cathy when she went on and on and it wasn't clear how it related to her goal," the supervisor should say, "When Cathy was going on and on about something that wasn't clearly related to her goal, I would interrupt and say that I wasn't understanding how this information was connected to the goal you've set for yourself, and it's really important that I understand this so that I can be as helpful to you as possible."

FORMAT FOR SUPERVISION

In order to be effective, supervision of the TRG should occur on a regular and reliable basis. We have found that 1 hour of weekly supervision beginning in the preparatory phase is needed by clinicians who are conducting this group for the first time. An hour of supervision every other week may be sufficient for clinicians who have conducted the group previously. The frequency of supervisory meetings may vary, depending on the phase of the group, as the co-leaders' needs may change over time. Although the needs for supervision may also vary, what never changes is the need for the co-leaders to take sufficient time to debrief each other, plan for the next session, and communicate about how they can best support each other in running the group.

The structure and content of supervision will also vary according to the group phase, co-leaders' needs, and the style of the supervisor. However, it is important that three areas be addressed in each supervisory session: (1) general observations about the group process, (2) individual member goals and problems, and (3) co-leaders' reactions to the group and their co-leadership. Given these multiple priorities, judicious time management is essential for supervision to be effective, paralleling the need for accurate time keeping within the group. We recommended that following each group session co-leaders consult with each other about the most important issues to be addressed in supervision and that the supervisor inquire about these issues at the start of the meetings. The Co-Leader's Group Tracking Notes for Supervisory meetings (provided in Appendix G) are designed to help co-leaders track individual members' progress and group process and to identify other topics to be discussed further in supervisory meetings. A completed sample is shown in Figure 7.1.

Since there is usually a lot of material to be discussed in these meetings, we recommend that the supervisor take good notes to reduce the need for repetition in subsequent

Date: May 5, 2009

Session number   6   of   16

Who took goal-work time in this group session? Lenore, Andrea, Sarah

Summarize the goal work and the feedback for each member who used time during this session. Pay close attention to goal development and the content of the feedback and its source.

Sarah: Working on ways to maintain emotional safety at brother's wedding in 3 weeks. Today practiced how to talk with people she is relying on for support about what she needs. Open to and received excellent feedback. Did role play with offer from Jill.

Andrea: Reports noticing a lot of shame as she is working on goal of writing her graduate school applications; feels she does not deserve to be admitted, judges her writing very negatively. Reports intrusive memories of harsh criticism from mother. Shared related traumatic memories. Susan asked about how she felt about what she had shared. Andrea connected with grief in acknowledging the origins of her shame and increased awareness of how limiting it has been in her life.

Lenore: STUCK!!! Went last after two members who are coming along well in regard to their goals. Expressed harsh self-criticism about challenges in defining her goal further: wants to feel connected to group. Members offered encouragement; however, Lenore had difficulty taking this in. HELP!!! We feel stuck, too, wanting to rescue Lenore. She is so good at being patient and supportive in her feedback to others. We understand her constant self-criticism and rejection of positive feedback as a way of maintaining distance from others. How can we communicate this observation to her without shaming her?

What interpersonal dynamics are evolving and/or are foreseeable in this group?

Concern that members will stop giving Lenore feedback because she tends to be dismissive. She may fall deeper into feeling stuck, especially given that other members on her time-taking week are progressing well toward their goals. Concerned that Lenore may sense our feeling stuck, too.

Maura was quite withdrawn today, same as last week. She says that she is preoccupied with problems she is having with her son, who has been discharged from his residential program.

What specific concerns or questions need to be discussed in supervisory meetings?

Need help with Lenore: defining goal, managing our countertransference, minimizing negative impact of group dynamics.

How to engage Maura and maybe tie her concerns about her son with goal of being able to practice asking for help.

Which members are taking goal-work time during the next session? What are the related questions or concerns?

Rose, Maura, Jill

If Rose continues to push time boundaries, how should we handle this? We reiterated reasons for the structure in a general way last session.

What co-leadership considerations or difficulties need to be discussed in supervisory meetings?

Countertransference, mentioned above. We both feel this way.

FIGURE 7.1. Example of completed Co-leader's Group Tracking Notes for Supervisory Meetings.

sessions. The Supervisor's Tracking Tool (see Appendix J) helps supervisors to summarize and track the work of each group member. A sample completed form for a TRG supervisory session is presented in Figure 7.2. At the beginning of the session, the supervisor and group co-leaders develop an agenda identifying the most important issues to be addressed, since temptations to deal with interesting but less urgent matters may sometimes intrude, thereby confusing priorities. Topics should be prioritized to ensure that the co-leaders depart with as many of their key concerns addressed as possible.

SUPERVISION OVER THE COURSE OF THE TRG

In addition to the general guidelines mentioned above, each phase of the TRG presents particular issues and challenges that should be addressed in supervision.

Preparatory Phase

It is important that supervisory arrangements be made before the co-leaders begin the screening process, as there is a lot of information to cover and it is important to stay up to date with the progress of the group. Starting supervisory meetings during the preparatory phase is especially important for co-leaders who are conducting this group for the first time. The supervisor can have an important role in orienting new group leaders to the group model. Once the co-leaders and supervisor have thoroughly read the treatment guide, supervisory sessions should be used to review the six key features of TRG therapy and to discuss any questions that may have arisen.

The supervisor can also advise the co-leaders with regard to planning for the group, considering such factors as time issues and duration of the therapy as well as potential local referral sources and member recruitment strategies. In preparing for the next phase, the supervisor should review the screening criteria with the co-leaders as well as the various components of the screening process. The supervisor can help to ensure that the leaders remain realistic in their planning, for example, by anticipating that the group intake process may take longer than initially expected.

The supervisor should also speak with the co-leaders about the purpose of supervision and encourage them to raise clinical dilemmas or unexpected personal reactions to members' interactions. He or she should also explicitly invite them to talk about co-leadership dynamics and address any power differentials between them (e.g., staff member vs. trainee). By recognizing these issues in advance rather than waiting for them to emerge on their own, the supervisor actively fosters a climate in which such issues can be openly discussed and ensures that power relations between the co-leaders are handled in way that is productive rather than destructive for the dyad and the group.

A list of pregroup preparation tasks was provided in Chapter 3 (in Table 3.1). The supervisor and group co-leaders can use this list collaboratively to identify and organize what needs to be done prior to beginning the group. Discussion of the initial therapist prepara-

Member's name: _Lenore_

Relevant history:

25 years old, Jewish heritage. Lives with roommate. Working as a temp. Mother active alcoholic during her childhood but now in recovery. Describes father in idealized way but also says he was highly critical/ had high expectations of her. Raped at age 18 by a "friend of a friend" after a party.

Individual therapy for 3 years, some trauma focus, recent content related to feeling stuck/ disconnected in the world.

Positive relationship with therapist who referred her to this group.

No current risk factors (past suicidal ideation but not during last few years), no hospitalizations, no medications.

Goal tracking (including process of operationalizing goal and any changes during group sessions):

trauma-related ____   present-oriented ____   achievable ____   concrete ____   specific ____

All aspects of above appear to be THE work for this patient initially.

Initial: Expressed difficulty in identifying and following though with a goal because of fear of disappointment and self-doubt, which make her feel stuck. Appears motivated to address this and understands goal requirement of group.

Session 2: Wants to feel connected to the group. Notes she feels superior sometimes, as a defense against feeling unloved. Supervision discussion today focused on how to operationalize this goal—ask how she would know this is happening. Also discussed how much to use group process and decided that it would be best not to encourage relational processing about feeling superior, but rather to take opportunities as they arise to note when others are relating in a caring way and help Lenore to notice when this is happening and what it feels like for her. Focusing on feeling superior would potentially be upsetting or silencing for other members.

Sessions 4/6: Lenore continues to offer VERY accurate empathetic feedback but remains vague on her own goal as well as very self-critical. Co-leaders feeling stuck as to how to help operationalize her goal, as Lenore's difficulty with this task is also becoming a source of self-criticism for her. Discussed use of feedback to Lenore regarding her empathy toward others and her difficulty in feeling any compassion for herself as well as in taking in feedback. Encouraged co-leaders to be very active in seeking responses from Lenore regarding her reactions to empathic feedback from others.

Session 8: Lenore reveals that a man who had taken her in after running away had lured her into prostitution. She states that she has never talked about it to anyone (not disclosed in intake). Is able to tell group that she feels "dirty and disgusting." Co-leaders responded effectively in both offering sociopolitical framework regarding prostitution, in order to help reduce shame.

Group members responded with an outpouring of support for her bravery. After significant feedback from others, co-leader asked what it was like to tell her story. For the first time, Lenore does not discredit feedback! Although goal still has not been fully articulated, ways to do so are becoming clearer. Co-leaders explore ways to use this experience in helping Lenore explain and explore her feelings of connectedness with the group.

Sessions 10/12: Doing well. Able to articulate feeling connected and reports a decrease in self-criticism. She is experimenting with risking more disclosure in outside relationships. Goal has not been specified; discussed importance of this task in order for Lenore to fully experience the mastery she is achieving.

(cont.)

FIGURE 7.2. Example of completed Supervisor's Tracking Tool.

Session 14: Lenore describes the changes she feels in being more connected through the process of sharing more of herself with the group. Co-leader steps in to help Lenore notice that she is describing the accomplishment of her original goal of feeling more connected, suggesting that she is able to both experience and describe what this means to her.

Participation (sharing/feedback etc.): Active participant, naturally able to provide empathetic and encouraging feedback to others. No problems regarding time taking, remaining focused. Process of receiving feedback is crucial to goal work, above.

Concluding session feedback: Lenore will get recommendation to continue consolidating and practicing her new skills. Ongoing use of individual therapy recommended. Group appears to have moved client out of a stuck place, needs opportunity to build on this momentum with new challenges, which will arise.

FIGURE 7.2. *(cont.)*

tion questions can be a helpful way to begin the supervisory relationship and for the supervisor to understand the learning needs and hopes of the group co-leaders.

Screening

During the screening phase, the supervisor's primary role is to help group leaders determine whether the group would be a good match for each potential client (based on the criteria described in Chapter 3) and to identify when more information should be sought out (e.g., through the referring therapist or by inviting the client to return for a second interview) in order to determine inclusion. Co-leaders should use this opportunity to provide the supervisor with sufficient background information about each potential group member so that the supervisor is well versed on members' particular circumstances even before the group begins its sessions. The supervisor should record this historical data for each client by using the Supervisor's Tracking Tool in Appendix J (discussed earlier and illustrated in Figure 7.2). The supervisor should pay close attention to the overall composition of the group, engaging the co-leaders in thinking about how each client fits in with the others as well as when and how to address areas of difference (taking into account the considerations noted in Chapter 3).

The screening phase is a useful time to begin talking about goal formulation in supervisory sessions, even if clients' stated goals change by the start of the group. The supervisor should use the information presented from in-take interviews to review with the co-leaders the criteria for evaluating clients' suitable goals for the TRG (i.e., that they be present-oriented, trauma-related, achievable, concrete, and specific). This process better equips co-leaders to help clients hone in on appropriate goals during the introductory phase of the therapy.

The supervisor's role during the screening phase is, in essence, to be "the voice of reason." One step removed from the group, he or she is less easily influenced by the personal and/or systemic pressures experienced by co-leaders to get the group started or by countertransference reactions that may affect decisions about group membership. The desire to get the group started is often accompanied by a willingness on the part of the group leaders to accept someone whose readiness or fit for the group is questionable. For example, one supervisor had to take a firm position against the admission of a client who had disclosed how her medical complications forced her to cancel many therapy sessions. She was hopeful that she would not need to do this during the course of the therapy, and the co-leaders felt guilty about denying membership to someone who so clearly could benefit from being in the group and whose physical complaints were also tied to her trauma. The supervisor, however, was convinced that accepting the client into the group was a "set-up" for failure, since her likely absences would only cause her to feel more isolated and "different" from other group members and therefore impede developing the relationships she craved. Hence, "making an exception" in this instance was not in the client's best interest. From his or her more objective vantage point, the supervisor can draw co-leaders' attention to issues that they may have overlooked. In another case, co-leaders mentioned that the prospective member had thought a lot about what it might entail for her to speak openly about her experiences and seemed caught off-guard when asked what it might be like to hear others' stories. The co-leaders liked her and felt that she was otherwise a good fit, and they were inclined to accept her. The supervisor suggested that co-leaders meet with the client again to discuss the issue further after she had had some time to consider the question they had earlier posed to her.

Another important function of the supervisor during the screening phase is to help the group leaders think about how to, in a gentle and constructive way, turn down a client who does not meet one or more important criteria for inclusion in the group. Co-leaders can be coached to help the client understand that this is just not a good time in her recovery process to participate in this particular group model, and to be clear and transparent about the reasons. Thus, the screening interview becomes a consultation where the client can benefit from a recommendation as to when this group might be appropriate. The use of role play can be helpful in preparing group leaders for this task, as it can also later in the therapy when co-leaders may be required to give difficult feedback. Clinicians and supervisors are referred to Chapter 3 for additional details on giving feedback from the screening interview.

Co-leaders immediately need to be in touch with clients who have been previously accepted if for any reason the group is unable to start on time. Supervisors can help leaders deal with clients' frustration while "on hold," perhaps suggesting ways their time can be used for continued preparatory work.

During the screening phase, the group co-leaders and supervisor collect a tremendous amount of information from clients and their collateral contacts and also consider how the group is developing as a whole. The information-gathering tools referenced and illustrated in this chapter may be particularly helpful in facilitating supervision during this phase.

Introductory Sessions

The supervisor's role during the introductory sessions is to support group leaders in establishing a sense of safety in the group and to help them accomplish the assigned tasks of the early sessions (as described in Chapter 4). Working with each member to define a present-oriented goal that can be clearly tied to her trauma history is a particularly important focus of supervision during this phase of TRG therapy. Although group members typically share a lot of information about themselves and their background, it is not essential that the supervisor know every detail about every client. Instead, co-leaders should be encouraged to focus on sharing with the supervisor whatever is most relevant about each client's goal and its relation to her trauma history. Building on the groundwork accomplished during the screening phase, the feedback from the supervisor should be directed at helping each group member make her goal more specific, concrete, and achievable. Throughout all stages of supervision, the supervisor should encourage co-leaders to take notes immediately after each group session.

The supervisor should be checking in with co-leaders about any salient group process issues that are emerging early during the therapy. Difficulties in time keeping (e.g., too prolonged an opening round, insufficient time for feedback, ending too late) should be addressed immediately. For many clinicians, the process of interrupting clients and redirecting them to share information that is relevant to the goal is the most challenging part of running this group. Often the issue is framed as "How can I silence people who have long been silenced by others, or have silenced themselves, all their lives? They finally get to a place where it is safe to share their trauma, and I have to interrupt constantly or say it's too early in the sessions to share details. How can that be therapeutic?" To respond effectively to this question the supervisor must believe that achieving one's goal and the accompanying sense of mastery that this experience provides are crucial to the recovery process and that they are contingent on adherence to the TRG treatment model. He or she must be prepared with concrete examples of how to intervene in a way that is firm, clear, and caring. Some examples of how to do so can be found in Chapter 4. It is important that the supervisor fully appreciate that many clinicians new to this type of therapy believe that their willingness to listen and be supportive is their biggest asset to clients. Therefore, until they feel they have developed a new skill set, they may be reluctant to shift from that stance. Members of the TRG typically come from families that have few boundaries and are either overly strict or negligent. For treatment to be successful, the therapist must be willing to set limits, redirect clients, and teach members the way to participate effectively in this group context. This approach will ultimately enhance group members' sense of accomplishment if it is carried out in a respectful and nonshaming manner. The supervisor should firmly believe that acquiring these new skills is both possible and that doing so will ultimately benefit the clients.

The supervisor should also ask about how well the co-leaders are working together. It is particularly important that *both* co-leaders make their presence felt during the early sessions, especially if one co-leader is more junior or was less involved in the screening process. The supervisor may need to advise the co-leadership pair on how to make this person's role more prominent (e.g., having her speak first or provide a more substantial portion of the orientation information). It is very important to have the junior clinician's voice heard during the earliest sessions, since establishing equal participation will only become more challenging a task as the group progresses. If the dominant leader does not step back and actively welcome this sense of equality, the resulting dynamic may prove distracting and upsetting to the members, as it replicates the relational patterns of domination and subordination with which many of them are familiar from their families of origin. This issue is even more crucial if the senior clinician is planning an absence during the course of the therapy, as the group will likely respond to the lack of leadership, for example, by caretaking the junior clinician (and protecting themselves) by holding back difficult material from her.

Goal-Work Sessions

During the goal-work phase, the supervisor's role is to assist the co-leaders in tracking each member's progress in relation to her goal and to plan interventions that may be helpful in moving members toward goal mastery. Whenever members' sharing seem unclear or unfocused, the supervisor should be asking how the member's use of her time (and the feedback that she is receiving) is connected with her goal and her trauma history—to prevent the group and co-leaders from becoming distracted by other issues. The supervisor may also need to help co-leaders realize when a member's goal needs to be reframed or modified in order to ensure a successful therapeutic experience. Just as it is useful to ask this question of group members, the supervisor should be asking group co-leaders how each client will know whether her goal has been achieved. By encouraging leaders to practice this style of thinking, he or she helps them to facilitate group members' development of this skill. The supervisor should remind group leaders when the midpoint of the group is approaching so that they in turn can remind the members. The Supervisor's Tracking Tool referenced earlier (see Appendix J) is designed to facilitate his or her focus on all of these tasks of supervision.

During this phase, the supervisor should be listening for common themes that may be emerging in the group and that can be referenced by co-leaders to promote cohesion. He or she should also be attending to the ways in which individual members' experiences may diverge from the more common themes and cause them to feel different or set apart from the group. Ultimately, it is helpful if group members can experience a blend of commonality and differentiation.

As was noted in Chapter 5, there is increased potential for interpersonal conflict during this phase of the TRG therapy. The supervisor plays a key role in helping co-leaders understand and decide how to respond to this conflict. If the interpersonal conflict presents an opportunity for members to deepen their goal-related work, the supervisor can help the co-leaders think about how to use the conflict productively. However, if the interpersonal conflict detracts from a member's goal work or threatens to derail the group, the supervisor can help the co-leaders find ways to contain or redirect it (e.g., by speaking with the member's individual therapist or meeting with the member outside of the group). It also sometimes happens that interpersonal conflict neither deepens nor detracts from members' pursuit of their goals but still needs to be addressed before the group can move on (e.g., some feedback has been misinterpreted). In this case, the supervisor can help co-leaders think about how to bring this issue back to the group to allow sufficient processing so that members can continue to do their work.

Again, the supervisor should be constantly monitoring co-leadership dynamics. There should be discussion about how the group appears to be reacting to the co-leaders, and co-leaders may need to adjust their position and levels of activity in the group in response to these observations. Any difficulties in co-leadership should be explored with a view to understanding the source of these problems and taking corrective action (e.g., Is the more experienced co-leader making it difficult for the junior co-leader to participate meaningfully? Does the more junior member need a greater familiarity with the treatment model?). Often a junior co-leader will state that it takes her time to plan what she wants to say, and by the time she has done that the co-leader has spoken. A concrete way to deal with that problem is for her to plan a response to a particular client or comment on a group process issue that has been discussed so that the clinician comes to the group prepared to deliver her feedback.

Not uncommonly, the supervisor of the TRG visits the group around the midpoint of treatment to obtain a more in-depth understanding of the group process, individual clients, and the co-leadership dynamics. When it happens, the group should be notified of the impending visit and its purpose as early as possible. To reduce clients' anxiety, the rationale for the visit should be clearly explained as the best way to help the co-leaders rather than represented as an evaluation of the group members' work. As noted earlier, during the visit the supervisor should sit outside of the group and share a few general observations toward the end of the session.

Toward the end of the goal-work phase, the supervisor should help group leaders think about any final steps that should be taken by members as they complete their goals. He or she should also encourage group leaders to remind members about the therapy's end date and to ask about reactions to the group's pending termination as this time approaches.

Concluding Sessions

Immediately prior to the concluding sessions, supervision should focus on ensuring that co-leaders understand and are able to explain the closing exercise (detailed in Chapter 6). There should be planning and discussion of specific feedback that the co-leaders will give to group members as well as of suggestions regarding "next steps." The supervisor should ask co-leaders to share responsibilities roughly equally in the final session so that each co-leader prepares feedback for half of the group's members. Prior to the final session, co-leaders share this work with each other (and their supervisor) so that additional observations can be incorporated.

In supervisory sessions, co-leaders should be provided with an opportunity to talk about their feelings about the end of the therapy. It has been our experience that co-leaders' feelings often mirror the feelings of relief, sadness, and accomplishment reported by group members. A final supervisory session should be scheduled to follow the conclusion of the group, thereby providing co-leaders an opportunity to review their experience of conducting the group and to supply final feedback to each other and the supervisor about their experience of working together.

CONCLUSION

Supervision is an essential requirement for TRG therapy to help leaders apply the treatment model, address clinical issues affecting individual members and the group as a whole, and feel supported in their difficult and demanding work. The experience of supervising the TRG bears many similarities to supervising other trauma-focused groups; however, it also entails an awareness and understanding of differences unique to this treatment model. While the supervisor's role is complex and challenging, it can ultimately be extremely rewarding to witness and facilitate the growth of the leaders and, indirectly, their group members.

CHAPTER 8

Adaptations and Applications

Although the TRG therapy model was initially developed for women survivors of childhood sexual abuse, the basic group model can be easily adapted to many other treatment populations. Because the model focuses on individualized goals, it permits great flexibility in its application. Unlike many other group treatments for trauma survivors, the TRG format is not dependent on specific presentations of psychoeducational material in weekly sessions. So long as its essential features are preserved, the model can be adapted quite readily satisfy the needs of diverse survivor groups.

ESSENTIAL ELEMENTS OF THE TRG

The TRG has six key elements that define its structure and should be maintained for the successful application of the treatment model. The reader is referred to Chapter 2 for an in-depth description of each of these features. Briefly, the TRG is *trauma-focused*, with group members generally expected to share parts of their trauma story with the group as a whole. It is *time-limited* in that it has well-defined starting and ending dates. It is *goal-oriented* in that each member's therapeutic work is guided by individualized goals, and formulating, tracking, and accomplishing these goals are the focal points of the group. It is structured by the technique of *time sharing*, which ensures equal participation of all members. It has a *supportive process*, with emphasis on learning to give and receive empathetic feedback rather than exploring group dynamics (unless these are immediately relevant to the member's goals). Finally, we strongly recommend *co-leadership* of the group as the ideal model. Although we would always recommend that the leader of any therapy group receive regular supervision or consultation, it becomes axiomatic whenever co-leaders are not a feasible alternative.

SCREENING CONSIDERATIONS

When considering adaptations to the basic TRG model, it is important to recall that this type of therapy is designed for survivors in Stage 2 of recovery. These are clients who have been able to achieve a reasonable degree of safety and basic self-care in their present lives and who feel emotionally ready to focus on telling their trauma story. Thus, regardless of the particular treatment group to which the model is applied, the criteria for participating should be consistent with those presented in Chapter 3. Potential group members must be physically safe; they must have some form of reliable ongoing social support; and they must have a sufficient repertoire of coping skills so that they are able to tolerate the intense emotions expressed within the sessions. Individuals with active psychosis or substance abuse should not participate in this type of group. Allowing exceptions to these key guidelines creates the risk of emotionally unsafe group experiences for *all* members.

Beyond these basic considerations, careful thinking must always be applied to the variety of participants that can be included in any one group. With careful screening, the TRG group model can help survivors to bridge differences in age, education, and social class; in fact, one of the most enlivening aspects of the group is its ability to bring together people from very diverse walks of life. However, as we pointed out in discussing screening, care should be taken to avoid a situation in which a group member is the "only one" of a particular demographic or subcategory.

Group leaders should have a thorough understanding of the broader sociopolitical and cultural context of the trauma population in question that can be brought to bear on decisions about inclusion. For example, in considering a TRG for war refugees and torture survivors, it would be unwise to include as members persons from opposing sides of a current or past conflict. The underlying sociopolitical issues would be too complicated to explore in a short-term group, and survivors from opposing sides might simply view one another as enemies. Similarly, members of a refugee community may be suspicious of one another based on class, religious, or political affiliations. These suspicions may or may not be well founded, but at a minimum they must be recognized and understood. These issues can best be managed by asking potential group members how they feel about participating in a group with people from their own country.

As a general rule, perpetrators of violence or abuse should never be included in the same group with victims. However, sometimes these distinctions become blurred: for example, some victims may have become perpetrators under duress or during an immature stage of development (or both, as for instance in the case of child soldiers). It is also true that some perpetrators have themselves been victims, though this is less common than is generally supposed (Herman, 1988). If the instances of perpetration are in the distant past and, most importantly, if the individual now feels remorse and does not rationalize or excuse his or her crimes, then an exception to the rule may be considered. The individual with a history of perpetration must then be prepared for the possibility that other group members will have negative reactions when this fact is first disclosed to the group. On the other hand, there is great potential for healing in the encounter between victims and perpetrators who are both really fellow victims and genuinely remorseful.

TWO ADAPTATIONS

The following adaptations to TRG treatment have been developed and implemented by us and our colleagues at the Victims of Violence (VOV) Program. We present them as a way of encouraging others to expand the range of applications of this therapy model to the many other groups of people who have been traumatized as the result of interpersonal violence. In the first example, an all-women's group is adapted to include both women and men. In the second example, a secular group is adapted to address issues within a particular religious community.

The "Co-Ed" Group

In the early stages of the women's movement, when women were speaking out about gender-based violence for the first time, survivor groups were restricted to women only. Later, when it became apparent that many men had also suffered childhood abuse, including sexual abuse, the initial response was to organize groups for men only. In each case, segregation by sex was related to the particular burden of shame carried by survivors.

While many survivors continue to prefer to participate in single-sex groups, others are open to the possibility of participating in mixed groups. We have chosen to present the "co-ed" group adaptation in some detail because it presents a more complicated challenge than a single-sex group. In order to develop this group model successfully, the modifications described below were required.

Co-leadership

Since we understand interpersonal trauma as resulting from abuse of power, a central tenet is to avoid replicating traditional gender roles and socially constructed power imbalances in choosing the co-leaders of this group. Therefore, whenever possible the group should be overseen by co-leaders of both sexes who can comfortably model a cooperative relationship. Differences in status and power that might exacerbate the gender differences should be consciously taken up and worked through by the co-leaders. For example, if a senior male clinician and a relatively less experienced female clinician are co-leading, special care must be taken to ensure that they both have an equal voice in the group. Although the female co-leader may be learning the model and the techniques of group leadership, she could take the lead in those parts of the early sessions that are less dependent on prior skill and knowledge, such as presenting the guidelines and leading the introductions exercise in Session 1. Throughout the therapy, she should be supported by her co-leader so that she does not automatically defer to him. Despite his greater experience, he and she should work together to make sure that she is viewed by group members as a powerful and competent co-leader in her own right. This model of co-leadership conveys to members the co-leaders' conscious intention to use power (in this case, of gender and seniority) safely and beneficially without necessarily denying actual differences. The supervisor should be skilled at noticing gender inequities even when they are relatively slight and unintentional. The steady attention to power dynamics throughout the group therapy is crucial in creating a safe environment where negotiations, disagreements, and differing views can be shared as they relate to group members' goals.

In the rare event that co-ed co-leadership is not feasible, the co-ed group can still be conducted successfully with one leader or even with two co-leaders of the same sex. Although gender power differentials may not be an issue between the co-leaders, they will of course be an inevitable component of the group experience. Inevitably the gender of the perpetrator influences clients' reactions to the gender of the group leaders. Most often, both men and women clients report histories of abuse by male perpetrators, but this is by no means *always* the case. Since both men and women are capable of abusing power, co-leaders should be sensitive to this issue and raise it directly when appropriate.

Screening

Co-leaders should make it clear to prospective members that the co-ed environment is likely to be a source of anxiety and curiosity for both men and women. They should also emphasize that participation in this kind of group is not an essential healing component for all survivors and that individual choice is essential in all recovery decisions. Checking in with oneself is often particularly difficult for trauma survivors who are affectively dissociated and thus may make decisions out of an eagerness to please or "do the right thing." When asked about co-ed group participation, men will often initially minimize their anxieties ("It's no big deal"), while many women will present with more overt anxiety ("I think the only man I will ever trust is my therapist—and sometimes I'm not sure about him"). Such reactions are a manifestation of socialized gender stereotypes, where men are limited to being seen as powerful and dangerous and are shamed into hiding their fears about being seen as the "weaker sex." These roles are needlessly constricting to both male and female survivors, as they often deepen shame for men and exacerbate fear for women.

Goals

The presence and feedback of opposite-sex survivors and the knowledge that all members share the experience of having survived abuse have implicit effects on the goal work for all group members. Some members may explicitly choose to utilize the presence of opposite-gender participants in establishing goals. For example, a male survivor might define his goal as telling a part of his trauma story in an affectively connected way to an audience that includes both men and women. A secondary goal for this participant might involve taking in empathetic feedback and caring from members of both sexes. Both men and women might choose as their goals determining from co-ed group members when they can appropriately divulge their trauma history in a dating situation or, alternatively, how to recognize signs of abusive behavior in a prospective romantic partner.

Group Process

Co-leaders should strive to be very competent time keepers, as *equal time sharing*, inherent to the model, is a particularly important safety and modeling aspect of the co-ed group process. Given the almost automatic and unconscious tendency of women to become more reticent in a co-ed environment, the co-ed group may allow both men and women participants to experience equal sharing for the first time. Both men and women usually find such an experience surprising and exhilarating.

As one might expect, process varies tremendously, even as it remains contained by the *supportive* structure of the group. Factors influencing the internal development of the group include the number of members of each sex, their sexual orientation and identification, and age, education, and social class. In co-ed groups the presence of difference is evident from the outset in a highly charged way. Nevertheless, we have found that in this group context male members ultimately end up being regarded as fellow victims, rather than as perpetrators, accomplices, or bystanders. For both men and women, co-ed TRG therapy is an opportunity for members to move beyond gender stereotyping and relate to the opposite sex on the basis of members' common humanity.

Owing to the characteristics of the population that we serve, we have not yet conducted a TRG for male survivors only, although we do have experience in conducting other trauma groups for men. However, in a setting that serves a large population of men in the middle stages of recovery, we believe that the TRG could easily be adapted for male survivors alone. The basic outlines of the group would remain unchanged. The only modification we might recommend is that both co-leaders should be men. Exit interviews with clients of the VOV Program have indicated that many male survivors feel greater shame when a woman is present and are particularly reluctant to discuss the details of sexual encounters or sexual dysfunction in their presence. That said, it is important for group leaders to make it clear early on that they understand why male survivors might also have difficulty trusting male authority figures, and to review the data indicating that the majority of perpetrators who abuse boys are men in positions of power (Dube et al., 2005; Holmes & Slap, 1998).

Faith-Based Healing Group

Two common sequelae of trauma are disruptions in one's personal spiritual life and loss of connection to a religious or spiritual community (Janoff-Bulman, 1992). These consequences seem to be particularly evident among those who were abused in childhood by parents or other trusted authority figures. For example, a community study of women with histories of childhood abuse found that abused women were significantly more likely than others to repudiate their religious faith or convert to another religion (Herman, Russell, & Trocki, 1986). For some victims, the loss of one's religious attachments means the loss of a powerful resource for healing. This loss is compounded when members of the clergy are themselves implicated in crimes of violence or exploitation or when religious authorities appear to condone or excuse such crimes (Boston Globe Investigative Staff, 2002).

A faith-based group may afford some participants an opportunity to repair this kind of disconnection and to reclaim their membership in a functioning religious community. As an example, we describe an adaptation called the Jewish Healing Group, designed by Janet Yassen, a senior clinician at the VOV Program. The group was formed in response to requests from a number of Jewish women survivors who felt that their spiritual needs or longings were not adequately shared or understood in a secular psychotherapy group. The purpose of the group was to help members understand the impact of the traumas that they had suffered on their spiritual life and/or their practice of Judaism. Referral sources included community organizations and social service centers, the Jewish community, and individual therapists.

Screening Criteria

Participants sought out this group for various reasons, with two major themes emerging. Some participants sought to be healed by consciously reconnecting with their spiritual life. Others just hoped to feel less isolated when they participated in the rituals and practices of the religious community. At the screening interview for the initial pilot group, there were collaborative discussions with potential members about the leaders' plan to use ritual as a part of the group. Their intention was to safely expose members to Jewish ritual as a form of desensitization as well as an education in how to create one's own practices for healing. All of this planning was carefully described and discussed with potential participants. The issue of having a male rabbi co-leader was discussed as well, as is described in greater detail below.

Co-leadership

The Jewish Healing Group was co-facilitated by a female clinician experienced in the Jewish faith and practice and experienced in implementing and supervising the TRG and by a male rabbi who was dedicated to the cause of healing the psychological and spiritual harms caused by violence against women. The rabbi explained to potential group participants that he was open to addressing issues of power and that he welcomed criticism and suggestions. He offered various interpretations on how Judaism specifically opposes abuse in the family, and thus the experiences of abuse described by members were condemned by him both as a rabbi and a human being. As his co-leader was the experienced professional in the pair, he was dependent on her skill and guidance in defining the group structure, understanding process, and supporting members' goal work. Had the rabbi not been willing to fully share power or defer to a female co-leader in regard to her areas of expertise, he would not have been asked to co-lead the group. The co-leaders thus had different areas of specialized knowledge and skill but were able to work together collaboratively and in a manner that recognized their mutually complementary contributions to the group.

Some clergy have pastoral counseling education and share a common language with clinicians, but they generally lack specific training in psychological trauma. Therefore, if a similar faith-based group is to be co-led by a member of the clergy, it is crucially important for that person to have sufficient background knowledge of the impact of interpersonal violence. He or she should be willing to speak about and educate his or her congregation on issues of abuse in the community, including physical and sexual abuse of children, partners, and elders. Such clergy should publicly identify themselves as people of integrity to whom abuse can be reported and who are willing to act forcefully to protect community members. They should be thoroughly familiar with the resources and services available to survivors and be able to make appropriate referrals. The cleric's house of worship can itself become a valuable resource by providing space and accommodations to self-help groups and healing circles readily. Clerical group leaders have to have established sufficient critical distance themselves from authoritarian or oppressive religious practices so that they can acknowledge the ways that the religious community might itself have caused harm in the past. In all these ways, religious leaders can become and be seen as sources of support, willing to exercise their power to prevent further abuse from occurring.

Group Format Modifications

Modifications to the TRG treatment in this instance included the addition of religious ritual practices at the beginning and end of each group session, and at the termination of the therapy. These modifications better enabled group members to transition themselves from daily life routines to the trauma focus of the group. Each meeting began with a short reading from a Jewish source to provide inspiration. These readings, generally drawn from Jewish liturgy, sacred texts, rituals, or ceremonies and interpretations (including some by feminist authors) usually focused on such themes as peace, safety, and harmony. After the first three sessions, these readings were set to music, the familiar tunes often evoking memories in ways that were more powerful than the spoken word alone. The female co-leader chose and led this ritual, which was followed by the usual check-in that typically begins TRG sessions. The closing round also included a song, first with words only but in later sessions with accompanying music.

Another modification was the inclusion of psychoeducation about various religious issues that were relevant to members' goal work. This material was provided chiefly by the rabbi, relating to topics of real significance to members. For example, issues of forgiveness arose frequently—forgiving self, forgiveness in the eyes of God, and forgiving others. Group members sometimes wondered what to do in the event that a former perpetrator asked for forgiveness and, too, how they should deal with the commandment to honor a father and mother who, in their case, had been abusive and neglectful. The question of communal responsibility for abuse was addressed as well as other theological questions related to creating meaning from one's traumatic experiences.

The final modification in the TRG format was a group visit to a synagogue, the idea originating in a particular group member's goal to "reclaim the space." Other group members were intrigued by the idea and offered to go along on the visit to witness this event.

Finally, all the group members decided that they would devote one whole session to the visit, with the visit taking place 2 weeks prior to the final group meeting. On the appointed day, members met at the synagogue office and entered the space together. No services were being conducted at the time, and the synagogue was empty. Those who had personal goals, such as being able to touch the Torah, were able to carry them out while others watched. The leaders led the group in a short prayer of gratitude and a song to wish one another healing. The entire visit was quite brief—about 45 minutes. Group members took some time during the following TRG session to process their reactions. In general, this house of worship adaptation was so well received that the group leaders recommended incorporating it into the general format of any faith-based TRG group. As Ms. Yassen summarized the experience: "Like any field trip, it was enlivening. And it turned out to be very useful for people, even if it was not directly related to everyone's goal. For those who wanted to find their way back to a congregation, the visit created a little community of healing. It deepened the sense of meaning that people found in their faith."

Goals

Some goals were similar to those described in earlier chapters of this volume, such as disclosure to a family member or preparing to attend a family get-together where a perpetrator would be present. A common theme in the goal work was the wish to take a concrete step in building a bridge back to their lost sense of religious community. For example, some group members had been abused by relatives who were active participants in a temple or synagogue. The fact that the perpetrators continued to be seen as pillars of a faith community was profoundly alienating to the victims. Group support helped these members differentiate between the fallibility of a particular person and/or congregation and the more enduring and trustworthy aspects of the religious community.

One member's goal involved signing up for a Jewish adult education class to feel more knowledgeable and comfortable with religious observance that she that she had long avoided, owing to its traumatic associations. One parent wanted to be able to attend religious school events with her children and not feel consumed by traumatic memories. Another woman who had dissociated during her religious education due to abuse that was going on at the time wanted to learn Hebrew again so that she could participate in services.

In summary, this adaptation, which arose from the needs of a faith-based community, appeared to be helpful in restoring group members to a sense of religious community and spiritual practice. While this particular example involved the Jewish faith, we suggest that this kind of adaptation might be suitable to members of many religious groups.

Because the VOV Program serves a multiply traumatized client population (with childhood abuse as the predominant trauma type), the two adaptation examples we have offered both involved this type of trauma. However, we varied the demographics of the afflicted population to encompass both genders in the first instance and a particular religious group in the second. In a similar fashion, the TRG therapy model could be adapted to other specific demographics such as age (e.g., adolescents), race, or native language and cultural background. By the same token, the therapy could be adapted to survivors of many other types of trauma. The model would be equally useful to such groups as torture survivors, political asylum seekers, veterans, and many other victims of interpersonal violence. Caregivers suffering from secondary traumatic stress could also benefit from an adapted model. Stigmatized populations that might also benefit from the TRG model include those with particular legacy burdens, such as Native Americans, Holocaust survivors, and their children. Victims of hate crimes, who have been targeted because of race, or others marginalized in the GLBT (gay, lesbian, bisexual, transgender) communities might also find the model useful.

Needs assessment for particular survivor groups can sometimes be conducted by means of a daylong workshop offered to the target population that includes some didactic presentations about trauma and that also offers the chance for members of a particular survivor group to meet, interact, and make their voices and their wishes heard. When considering an adaptation to a particular survivor grouping, leaders should be familiar with the social ecology and the daily life experiences of the group in question. For example, if TRG therapy is adapted for combat veterans with war trauma, the group leaders should have a basic familiarity with the details of a soldier's life in the theater of war. It is not necessary—though it might be beneficial—for the group leaders to be combat veterans themselves. What gives the group leaders credibility, beyond their professional understanding of the effects of interpersonal violence, is their commitment and dedication to serving the particular survivor group in question. Survivors are usually very good judges of those qualities.

CONCLUSION

This chapter presents two adaptations of the TRG, a co-ed group and a faith-based healing group. This same model can serve as a template that practitioners working with other traumatized populations can modify to meet the needs of their clients. Group leaders should be familiar with the theory behind the model, adhere to the screening guidelines, and maintain the integrity of the six key elements. With these considerations in mind, the TRG model can be adapted successfully to a diverse range of trauma survivors.

CHAPTER 9

Outcome Research
on the Trauma Recovery Group

At the VOV Program of the Cambridge Health Alliance, where the TRG has been implemented as part of a comprehensive group therapy program, we have been systematically
collecting quantitative and qualitative outcome data from clients participating in these and
other groups. This study has been largely naturalistic; clinical and ethical considerations at
our site have precluded use of a wait-list comparison group, and the stage-based treatment
model is inconsistent with random assignment of clients to the TRG or other groups offered
at our program for clients earlier in recovery. All of the research described in this chapter
was approved by the Cambridge Health Alliance Institutional Review Board.

QUANTITATIVE FINDINGS

Study 1

The first study is a naturalistic study investigating the nature of changes reported by participants over the course of the TRG. As has been noted earlier, PTSD symptoms and depression
are the most commonly investigated outcomes in the literature on group therapy for trauma
survivors, although some studies also include measures of dissociation, self-esteem, anxiety, fear, and "global distress" (Foy et al., 2000). This study sought to broaden the range of
outcomes investigated to include changes in core processes associated with complex PTSD,
including emotional regulation, core beliefs about self, and interpersonal functioning. These
domains are more frequently the target of TRG goals than symptomatic change, since group
members would normally have stabilized and achieved some measure of symptom management stability prior to participating in a Stage 2 group. It is therefore particularly important

that they be represented in an outcomes assessment. We hypothesized that, in addition to any symptomatic changes exhibited by TRG participants, they would also show significant improvements in self-esteem and core schemas about self, affect regulation, and interpersonal functioning.

Method

SAMPLE

The sample consisted of 50 women who enrolled in successive iterations of the TRG. The groups averaged 21 weeks in length, with a range of 16–32 weeks. Follow-up data are available for 43 participants, 86% of those who began the group treatment. This retention rate compares very favorably with other group therapy studies (Yalom & Leszcz, 2005) as well as trauma treatment outcome studies (Schottenbauer, Glass, Arnkoff, Tendick, & Gray, 2008). It should be noted, however, that fewer data are available for the measures of affect regulation, core schemas, and interpersonal functioning, as these were added later in the overall study.

Participants ranged in age from 26 to 62 years, with a mean of 42.72 (SD = 10.57) years. The vast majority of the sample (78%) were European American; other groups represented in small numbers included African American, Asian American, and Native American participants. Some 76% were employed in some capacity, 15% were receiving disability, and 9% reported having no income. Some 46% were single, 26% were married or partnered, 18% were divorced, and 4% were widowed.

Of the sample, 96% were receiving concurrent individual therapy, and 74% were receiving psychopharmacological treatment at the VOV Program or elsewhere. Some 78% had a clinician-assigned diagnosis of PTSD, and 38% had a clinician-assigned diagnosis of major depression; 54% had two or more comorbid diagnoses. The mean global assessment of functioning (GAF) score for participants was 62.65.

Trauma history information is available for a subset of participants (n = 23). As can be seen in Table 9.1, the majority reported having experienced interpersonal violence by a known perpetrator. The mean number of different traumatic events reported by participants was 6.30 (SD = 2.48). The vast majority (96%) reported that the event causing them the most distress occurred more than 5 years earlier, 80% reported that it occurred before the age of 18 years, and 65% reported that it occurred over a number of years.

MEASURES

Posttraumatic Stress Diagnostic Scale. The Posttraumatic Stress Diagnostic Scale (PDS; Foa, Cashman, Jaycox, & Perry, 1997) is a 49-item self-report instrument designed to aid in the diagnosis of PTSD, with its structure and content mirroring the DSM-IV PTSD diagnostic criteria. It includes a checklist of possible traumatic events. We used the PDS's Symptom Severity score in these analyses to assess severity levels of the participants' PTSD symptoms. This score is based on 17 items assessing the frequency of posttraumatic stress

TABLE 9.1. Trauma Exposure among TRG Participants

Interpersonal trauma type	Frequency (%)
Adulthood	
Physical assault/stranger	8 (35%)
Physical assault/known person	9 (40%)
Sexual assault/stranger	5 (22%)
Sexual assault/known person	10 (44%)
Childhood	
Physical abuse/stranger	1 (5%)
Physical abuse/acquaintance	3 (15%)
Physical abuse/family	13 (65%)
Sexual abuse/stranger	1 (5%)
Sexual abuse/acquaintance	7 (33%)
Sexual abuse/family	8 (38%)
Physical neglect	13 (59%)
Emotional abuse	20 (87%)

symptoms on a scale of 0–3, with a total possible score of 51. According to the norms published in the manual, individuals with a diagnosis of PTSD obtain a mean score of 33.59, whereas individuals without this diagnosis score around 23.41. The developers (Foa et al., 1997) further designate scores of less than 10 as "mild," between 11 and 20 as "moderate," between 21 and 35 as "moderate to severe," and 36 and above as "severe." The PDS has demonstrated good sensitivity and specificity, internal consistency and test–retest reliability, and concurrent and convergent validity.

Beck Depression Inventory. The Beck Depression Inventory (BDI; Beck, Ward, Mendelson, Mock, & Erbaugh, 1961) is an extensively used inventory designed to assess the current severity of depression that was developed from clinical observations of depressed and nondepressed psychiatric clients. Attitudes and symptoms consistent with depression are represented in a 21-item questionnaire, and clients are asked to rate the severity of each on an ordinal scale of 0–3. A total score on the BDI is obtained by summing the ratings, with higher scores indicating greater depressive symptomatology. The following ranges have typically been used to guide decision making in clinical and research settings: 0–9, absent or minimal depression; 10–18, mild to moderate depression; 19–29, moderate to severe depression; and 30–63, severe depression. The BDI displays high internal consistency as well as good concurrent validity and construct validity (Beck, Steer, & Garbin, 1988).

Dissociative Experiences Scale. The Dissociative Experiences Scale (DES; Bernstein & Putnam, 1986) is a commonly used 28-item self-report questionnaire developed to assess dissociation in normal and clinical populations. Respondents indicate the percentage of the time they experience particular dissociative phenomena on a scale of 0–100% of the time. The overall DES score is based on the mean of all individual item scores, such that the DES total score can range from 0 to 100. A cutoff of 30 is frequently used to screen clients at high risk for dissociative disorders (Carlson & Putnam, 1993). A meta-analytic study of the DES revealed high internal consistency and good test–retest reliability, with excellent convergent and predictive validity (van IJzendoorn & Schuengel, 1996).

Rosenberg Self-Esteem Survey. The Rosenberg Self-Esteem Survey (RSES; Rosenberg, 1965) is a very commonly used measure of global self-esteem. It consists of 10 items answered on a 4-point scale ranging from "strongly agree" to "strongly disagree." The measure consists of an equal number of positively and negatively worded items. When negatively phrased items are reversed and responses are scored from 1 to 4, this procedure creates a scale ranging from 10 to 40, with higher scores indicating better self-esteem. A recent international study of the measure found a mean score of 32.21 ($SD = 5.01$) among U.S. participants (Schmitt & Allik, 2005). The RSES has been extensively studied and demonstrates acceptable internal consistency and test–retest reliability, as well as convergent and discriminant validity (Blascovich & Tomaka, 1991).

Schema Questionnaire—Short Form. The Schema Questionnaire—Short Form (SQ-S2; Young & Brown, 2003) is a shortened form of the Schema Questionnaire developed to assess early maladaptive cognitive schemas. It consists of 75 items selected to represent 15 maladaptive schemas. Participants rate how well each item describes them on a 6-point scale. Higher scores indicate a greater presence of that maladaptive schema in the respondent. We used an overall mean schema score for the purpose of these analyses. A factor analytic study provided strong support for the construct validity of the SQ-S2 and indicated that the subscales have adequate to very good internal consistency (Welburn, Coristine, Dagg, Pontefract, & Jordan, 2002).

Inventory of Interpersonal Problems. The Inventory of Interpersonal Problems (IIP-32; Barkham, Hardy, & Startup, 1996) is a shortened version of the Inventory of Interpersonal Problems (Horowitz, Rosenberg, Baer, Ureno, & Villasenor, 1988), which was designed to measure interpersonal distress experienced by psychiatric clients and evaluate change over the course of treatment. The items reflect a variety of interpersonal difficulties reported at intake by clients seeking outpatient psychotherapy, and comprise eight subscales. A total mean IIP-32 score was used in the current analyses. Horowitz et al. (1988) indicate that the original measure has good reliability, validity, and sensitivity to change, and the shorter version appears to sacrifice little in terms of the good reliability, validity, and sensitivity to change of the original measure (Barkham et al., 1996).

Difficulties in Emotion Regulation Scale. The Difficulties in Emotion Regulation Scale (DERS; Gratz & Roemer, 2004) is a 36-item measure of difficulties with various dimensions of emotion regulation. The scale provides a total score (used in the present study) as well as six subscale scores. Preliminary findings suggest that the DERS has high internal consistency, good test–retest reliability, and adequate construct validity and predictive validity (Gratz & Roemer, 2004).

PROCEDURE

At the start of the TRG, all participants were asked to complete a packet of the self-report measures described above. Clients were asked to complete an identical set of self-report questionnaires at the treatment's completion. The questionnaire packet took approximately 1 hour to complete, and additional clinical information (e.g., diagnosis, GAF score, current treatments) was collected from the group leaders. These self-report data are routinely collected from all clients participating in group treatment at the VOV Program; they are utilized for clinical purposes in treatment planning, and, with the clients' consent, they also contribute to a research database of group therapy outcomes.

Results and Discussion

We used dependent-samples t-tests to assess changes in scores on self-report measures from pre- to posttreatment. Cohen's d was computed for each analysis as a measure of effect size. The means and standard deviations are presented in Table 9.2.

Over the course of treatment, participants in the TRG demonstrated significant reductions in depression, $t(42) = 3.03$, $p < .01$, $d = .47$; posttraumatic stress, $t(39) = 2.84$, $p < .01$, $d = .46$; and dissociation, $t(42) = 2.07$, $p < .05$, $d = .32$. They also displayed significant improvements in self-esteem, $t(38) = -5.54$, $p < .01$, $d = -.88$, as well as reduction in interpersonal problems, $t(19) = 2.44$, $p < .05$, $d = .55$, and affect regulation difficulties, $t(19) = 2.15$, $p < .05$, $d = .48$. Only the measure of dysfunctional core beliefs did not reflect significant change, $t(19) = 1.72$, ns.

Given the threats to internal validity associated with the absence of a control or comparison group and random assignment, it is not possible to rule out the contribution of factors other than participation in the TRG to the observed improvements. Since participants' experience of trauma generally occurred in the remote past, and they were chronically

TABLE 9.2. Study I: TRG Descriptive Data

Measure	Pregroup		Postgroup		
	M	SD	M	SD	n
BDI	20.52	11.22	16.45	9.04	43
PDS	26.42	9.11	22.50	11.03	40
DES	16.85	10.29	14.67	9.86	43
RSES	23.50	5.08	26.13	5.15	39
SQ-S2	2.92	0.75	2.74	0.83	20
IIP-32	1.60	0.58	1.32	0.65	20
DERS	97.55	24.70	90.95	27.12	20

Note. Sample sizes vary, owing to the addition of new measures over time. BDI, Beck Depression Inventory; PDS, Posttraumatic Stress Diagnostic Scale; DES, Dissociative Experience Scale; RSES, Rosenberg Self-Esteem Scale; SQ-S2, Schema Questionnaire—Short Form; IIP-32, Inventory of Interpersonal Problems–32; DERS, Difficulties in Emotion Regulation Scale.

symptomatic, it is highly unlikely that time alone contributed to their improvement, espe-cially over the course of a 4- to 8-month group. Virtually all participants were receiving multimodal treatment with considerable variability in providers and treatment locations, and thus it is unlikely that other treatments produced any kind of systematic effect. Another potential criticism of these findings relates to the use of multiple *t*-tests, which can inflate family-wise error, increasing the likelihood of spurious findings. While this possibility can-not be disregarded, it important to note that effect sizes were generally in the moderate-to-large range, and significance was obtained with sample sizes as small as 20.

The lack of significance for the early maladaptive schemas represented by the SQ-S2 contrasts with the positive change obtained on related measures, especially on the RSES, which evidenced a very robust effect. These analyses were based on an overall mean score on the YSQ, which is composed of five domains and 15 schemas; it is likely more detailed evaluation would reveal changes on specific scales and domains.

Study 2

A number of clinical and ethical realities have made it difficult to conduct a randomized clinical trial of the TRG at our site. While our program offers clients in early recovery a variety of therapy groups aimed at safety, psychoeducation, and symptom management, the TRG (and a "co-ed group" based on the same treatment model) are the only groups oriented to clients later in recovery. We therefore do not have an existing appropriate comparison group to which we could randomize clients while remaining consistent with the principles of stage-based treatment. Clinical and administrative pressure to treat clients promptly and ethical concerns about withholding treatment from clients in need have argued against assigning some clients to a wait-list control group. The multitude of treaters and treatment combinations associated with our client population has rendered "treatment as usual" unhelpful as a source of comparison. All of these factors have frustrated researchers' efforts to study the efficacy of the TRG in a more rigorously scientific manner.

Although not ideal, one early recovery group offered at our program presents an opportunity for some comparison, as the clients it attracts have some diversity in regards to recovery stage. The Trauma Information Group (TIG) developed by Lois Glass and Bar-bara Hamm is a semimanualized group lasting 10–14 weeks that provides psychoeducation about the impact of trauma. In the group, which is present-focused, each session is orga-nized around a topic (e.g., trust, anger, remembering, shame and self-blame), and members are expressly discouraged from disclosing details about their trauma histories. While many clients referred to TIG are typical "early-recovery" clients who are highly symptomatic and just beginning to grapple with the meaning of a trauma-related diagnosis, there are others who are more stable but do not meet criteria for participation in a later recovery group such as the TRG for such reasons as having done little or no trauma work or having recently changed therapists. "Early recovery" thus characterizes the focus of the TIG but not neces-sarily the makeup of clients who participate in this group. As a result, there is a segment of these clients who may be an appropriate (albeit somewhat artificial) comparison group for the TRG.

The purpose of the TIG is to provide survivors with a cognitive framework for understanding their symptoms and a sense that they are not alone in their experiences, thereby promoting normalization and mastery and decreasing isolation. While these developments are likely to foster more positive feelings about the self, changing self-perception is not a primary focus of the group, and the group process is not utilized for this purpose. Indeed, the group is structured more like a seminar than a therapy group, which is very helpful in facilitating the engagement of more reluctant or fearful clients and those new to treatment. TRG treatment addresses trauma-related symptoms both through psychoeducation about trauma and its impact and the sharing of coping skills that occurs organically throughout the group, as well as the exposure component embedded in sharing the trauma narrative with the group in an affectively connected manner. We believe that TRG therapy targets survivors' self-esteem in a variety of ways:

1. The focus on formulating and achieving concrete goals provides members with a sense of personal agency and empowerment;
2. Clients are actively assisted in "hearing" and internalizing positive feedback received from others in the group;
3. Clients share memories and emotions that they have kept hidden and experience the acceptance and empathy of group members, which is a powerful antidote to feelings of shame and self-criticism; and
4. Clients develop respect for other group members with whom they can identify and are thereby challenged to address the dissonance between their perceptions of themselves and others.

Based on these characterizations of the two types of groups, we hypothesized that both TRG and comparable TIG members would demonstrate significant improvements in symptoms of PTSD, depression, and dissociation. We further hypothesized that TRG participants would show significantly greater improvements in self-esteem.

Method

SAMPLE

The sample in this study consisted of the 50 women described in the earlier cited study plus an additional 36 women who participated in the TIG and obtained initial scores on all three primary symptom measures discussed earlier (the PDS, BDI, and DES) within one standard deviation of the TRG participants. Independent-samples t-tests of initial scores on the measures of PTSD, depression, dissociation, and self-esteem confirmed that there were no significant pretreatment differences between participants from the two groups. Follow-up data on all four measures are available for 20 (56%) of the TIG participants as compared with 36 (72%) of the TRG participants. The relatively smaller proportion of TIG participants who completed follow-up packets likely results from the combination of higher dropout rates from early recovery groups and more focused data collection efforts on the TRG for purposes of developing this treatment guide.

Participants in the TIG had a mean age of 40.47 years (*SD* = 10.97). Some 63% were employed in some capacity, 27% were receiving disability, and 10% reported having no income. Some 48% were single, 30% were married or partnered, 19% were divorced, and 3% were widowed. European American participants constituted 71% of the sample, while 10% were African American and the remainder belonged to other groups or identified more than one ethnicity. There were no significant demographic differences between TRG participants and this subset of TIG participants.

TIG participants reported experiencing, on average, 8.33 (*SD* = 3.90) different types of traumatic events. Some 72% of TIG participants were receiving medications, and 93% were receiving concurrent individual therapy. There were no significant differences in trauma frequency or use of other treatment modalities between participants in the TIG and TRG.

Approximately 83% of TIG participants had a clinician-assigned diagnosis of PTSD, and 17% had a clinician-assigned diagnosis of major depression. Major depression was diagnosed significantly less frequently among TIG than TRG participants, $\xi^2 = 4.62, df = 1, p < .05$. Some 33% of TIG participants had two or more co-morbid clinician-assigned diagnoses, as compared with 54% of TRG participants; this difference was not statistically significant. The clinician-assigned GAF for TIG participants (*M* = 59.86, *SD* = 6.15) was significantly lower than for TRG participants (*M* = 62.65, *SD* = 4.64), with $t(67) = -2.15, p < .05$. These differences are likely more attributable to variations in the amount of clinical information gathered by clinicians during the intake process for the two types of groups rather than to real differences in clinical presentation. Since the TIG has fewer exclusion criteria, the screening process is considerably briefer and involves more limited history taking and diagnostic assessment.

MEASURES

The measures used in this analysis included the PDS, the BDI, the DES, and the RSES, all of which are described in detail earlier. The IIP-32, DERS, and SQ-SF were not included due to sample size limitations.

PROCEDURE

The procedures utilized in this study were identical to those in Study 1, described earlier.

Results and Discussion

We analyzed the data by using repeated measures multivariate analysis of variance (MANOVA). Means and standard deviations for the two groups are reported in Table 9.3. Repeated measures MANOVA revealed that participants in both groups made significant improvements from pre- to postgroup assessment on the measures of depression, $F(1, 54) = 7.58, p < .01, \eta_p^2 = .12$; posttraumatic stress, $F(1, 54) = 12.75, p < .01, \eta_p^2 = .19$; dissociation, $F(1, 54) = 6.58, p = .05, \eta_p^2 = .11$); and self-esteem, $F(1, 54) = 12.45, p < .01, \eta_p^2 = .19$. We found a significant interaction for type of group on the self-esteem (RSES) variable, with participants in the TRG making significantly more improvement in self-esteem over

TABLE 9.3. Study 2: Pre- and Postgroup Descriptive Data

Measure	Pregroup			Postgroup		
	TIG M (SD)	TRG M (SD)	Overall M (SD)	TIG M (SD)	TRG M (SD)	Overall M (SD)
BDI	18.22 (4.47)	20.79 (11.48)	19.87 (9.61)	15.44 (9.31)	16.18 (9.30)	15.92 (9.23)
PDS	26.50 (5.56)	26.53 (9.24)	26.52 (8.06)	21.58 (9.88)	22.10 (11.28)	21.91 (10.71)
DES	14.10 (5.88)	16.39 (10.71)	15.57 (9.28)	11.64 (6.73)	14.15 (10.07)	13.26 (9.04)
RSES	25.34 (4.35)	23.74 (5.15)	24.31 (4.90)	25.70 (4.99)	26.44 (5.16)	26.17 (5.07)

Note. TIG, Trauma Information Group; TRG, Trauma Recovery Group. For TIG, $n = 20$; for TRG, $n = 36$. BDI, Beck Depression Inventory; PDS, Posttraumatic Stress Diagnostic Scale; DES, Dissociative Experience Scale; RSES, Rosenberg Self-Esteem Scale.

the course of treatment than did participants in the TIG, $F(1, 54) = 7.26, p < .01, \eta_p^2 = .12$. This interaction is displayed in Figure 9.1. There were no significant interactions for type of group on the BDI, $F(1, 54) = .46, ns$; the PDS, $F(1, 54) = .03, ns$; or the DES, $F(1, 54) = .01, ns$; that is, members of the TIG and the TRG did not differ significantly in their amount of change in regard to these variables.

The results thus confirmed the hypothesis that, while participants in both groups would make comparable symptomatic improvements, TRG members would make signifi-

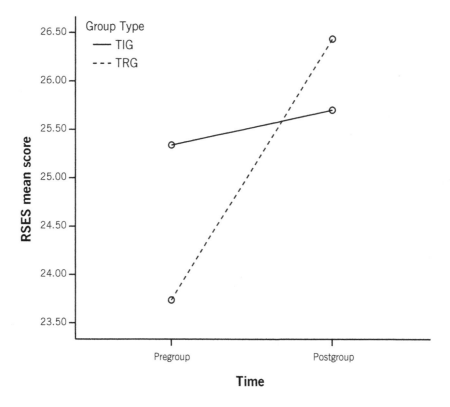

FIGURE 9.1. Group type and change in self-esteem.

cantly greater changes in self-esteem. The findings regarding self-esteem are important because impaired self-perception is a particularly pernicious long-term effect of prolonged exposure to interpersonal violence such as childhood abuse (e.g., Arata, Langhinrichsen-Rohling, Bowers, & O'Farrill-Swails, 2005) and domestic violence (e.g., Zlotnick, Johnson, & Kohn, 2006). There is some evidence of especially negative effects associated with emotional abuse that may accompany other forms of abuse or occur independently (Briere & Runtz, 1993; Finzi-Dottan & Karu, 2006).

This study is clearly limited by the use of a comparison group that was created retrospectively. Furthermore, the TIG (10–14 weeks) was shorter in duration than the TRG (16–32 weeks), which could have contributed to the results regarding self-esteem. It was also unfortunate that there were insufficient data available on early maladaptive schemas, interpersonal functioning, and affect regulation to include in the analyses. A redesigned study utilizing an appropriate control group and more detailed assessment of the important areas of impact would strengthen confidence in these findings.

Summary and Conclusions

These two quantitative studies provide preliminary evidence of the effectiveness of the TRG. Because this is a naturalistic study, the findings have ecological validity and generalizability to trauma survivor populations that are frequently seen in clinical practice. The absence of an appropriate control group, lack of randomization, and many sources of variability in a study of this nature make it impossible to rule out explanations other than group participation for the improvements observed among study participants. We hope that the availability of this treatment guide will facilitate further studies in diverse settings that will confirm and expand these findings.

The quantitative outcome data described above shed some initial light on the types of changes clients make when they receive treatment through use of the TRG model. Hearing participants express in their own words their experience of the TRG is an invaluable source of information about the specific and concrete ways in which this particular group model impacts their recovery. The next section describes the results of a narrative study of treatment outcomes among women participating in the TRG. We draw connections between the quantitative self-report data and narrative data to illustrate where the latter provide a greater amount of important context and depth in our understanding of the recovery process.

QUALITATIVE FINDINGS

Qualitative methods, broadly defined, are a growing area of interest in a number of disciplines and have begun to be of interest in psychology. Researchers, including those who study traumatic stress and dissociation, have been drawn to narrative and qualitative methods to understand individuals' accounts of their experiences in greater depth (Mishler, 2004). Survivors' narratives, as they make meaning of their experiences, have the capacity to demonstrate which factors may contribute most to change, which can in turn aid in the psychotherapy process. Further, qualitative methods permit a closer and more complex look at issues that may be hard to capture in self-report methods such as interpersonal dynamics and complex and at times contradictory coping mechanisms. The strength of qualitative research lies in its flexibility and ability to address these complex issues while including the participant as an active agent in the research process. Qualitative research methods are also particularly compatible with a feminist approach and an empowerment orientation, as survivors are encouraged to speak in their own words, and their voices are expressed through the narrative data (Reinharz, 1992).

As both qualitative and quantitative methods have their strengths and weaknesses, the integration of these methods can be extremely valuable in enhancing our understanding of trauma and recovery. Quantitative methods enable the researcher to gather larger and more anonymous amounts of information and also to collect demographic data that can be extremely useful. Owing to the sensitive nature of trauma-related material, anonymous questionnaires may be the best way to elicit certain information, as participants may feel less inhibited by the research process. Quantitative methods may thus reduce some of the artifacts inherent in such research (Cook & Campbell, 1979). However, Denzin and Lincoln (1998) point out that quantitative methods, in seeking the average across participants, may miss the complexity of each participant's unique perspective. Qualitative methods may be particularly helpful in redressing this problem, although they also have their particular limitations. Specifically, owing to the increased time required to perform this kind of research, we may be able to collect data only from a small group of participants, which in turn may raise questions about generalizability (Denzin & Lincoln, 1998). Therefore, only by using quantitative and qualitative methods together can we provide a more accurate picture of what is going on and increase our confidence in the research results.

Narrative Study

We now present the qualitative outcome data that we gathered from narrative interviews with TRG participants during the process of developing this treatment guide. We then consider their similarities and differences from the self-report data reported earlier in this chapter. As will be seen, some themes substantiate the quantitative findings, and others provide a different level of complexity in understanding the recovery process in this therapy group.

Method

SAMPLE

Six women who had participated in the TRG during the development of this treatment guide were interviewed after the therapy's completion. Five of the women were European American, and one was Asian American. Their ages ranged from 36 to 62. Four participants reported histories of childhood sexual abuse, and four also reported having experienced rape as an adolescent or an adult. Three participants noted histories of childhood physical abuse. All participants simultaneously were engaged in outpatient psychotherapy and received psychopharmacological treatment. The primary clinician-assigned diagnoses were either PTSD or major depression.

MEASURES

The Multidimensional Trauma Recovery and Resiliency Interview (MTRR-I; Harvey, Westen, Lebowitz, Saunders, Avi-Yonah, & Harney, 1994) is a semistructured interview that asks trauma survivors to talk about their history, experiences, relationships, and current functioning across eight domains of trauma recovery: (1) authority over memory, (2) integration of memory and affect, (3) affect tolerance and regulation, (4) symptom mastery and positive coping, (5) self-esteem, (6) self-cohesion, (7) safe attachment, and (8) meaning. Participants are also asked to describe their ability to manage their symptoms, their feelings about themselves, what has helped them cope, and their feelings about the future. The MTRR-1 has been translated into multiple languages and has multicultural utility for both treated and untreated survivors (Daigneault, Cyr & Tourigny, 2007; Peddle, 2007; Tummala-Narra, 2007). We modified the measure to focus on any changes respondents had noticed since their participation in the group, adding the following questions:

> What were your expectations and goals for the group?
> What was your experience in the group?
> What was most helpful about the group?
> What did you not find helpful about the group?
> How do you think the group treatment that you have received has affected
>   your recovery?
> What, if any, changes have resulted from your group participation?

PROCEDURE

All of the women participated in the quantitative studies described earlier in this chapter, completing self-report questionnaires before and after the group treatment. They also agreed to participate in an in-depth interview before and after the group. The data described here are derived from the postgroup interviews. We interviewed clients on site at the clinic and compensated them financially for their participation. Each interview was approximately 90–120 minutes in length and was audiotaped and transcribed.

We utilized a grounded theory approach (Strauss & Corbin, 1990) to analyze interview transcripts. Grounded theory is an inductive methodology intended to generate theory from narrative text coded into descriptive categories. Data are systematically coded and compared in order to generate conceptual categories and identify their properties as well as the relations among them (Creswell, 1998). In this way, the resulting theory should be meaningful and logically consistent because it is both grounded in and accountable to the data (Rennie, Phillips, & Quartro, 1988). We conducted a line-by-line analysis of each interview (a process called "microanalysis"). This microanalytical process contributed to the next stage in grounded theory analysis, called "open coding," the process of "breaking down, examining, comparing, conceptualizing, and categorizing data" (Strauss & Corbin, 1990, p. 61). We examined narratives as wholes, identified the significant and prevailing concepts, and discovered their properties and dimensions, which are presented below. The small number of participants in this study limits the generalizability of the qualitative results, but the voices of group members themselves provide an important perspective into the experience of this model of group treatment.

Results

Some broad themes emerged in the interviews that provided a considered and complex view, from the participants' perspective, of the benefits and challenges of this group model. The group enabled participants to combat their sense of isolation and alienation. Participation in the TRG helped them challenge and rework relational patterns and schemas and enabled them to begin rebuilding their relational capacities. Members developed an understanding of the more subtle aspects of trauma and how it affected their lives. This issue was especially relevant because the group is designed for members who have typically done a significant amount of work on reducing their trauma symptoms and are hoping to address more complex and unyielding problems in their experience of themselves and their relationships. Finally, participants also referred to symptomatic and concrete changes that occurred over the course of the therapy. As we illustrate below, these themes echo many of the self-report findings but also extend them to provide a uniquely complex view of the interpersonal aspects of the group and how such interactions enabled members to achieve their goals.

1. The first important theme that emerged in the interviews was that the group enabled participants to combat their sense of isolation and alienation. Through the witnessing that the women offered one another in the group context, participants felt that their sense of shame, stigma, and secrecy diminished as well as their tendency to minimize their trauma. By connecting with other trauma survivors in a safe environment and sharing their experiences, they received empathy, support, kindness, and a sense of belonging in return. These benefits were expressed in many different ways:

> "I liked it [the group] very much. I felt that ease to be able to share my experiences with other women, and it was kind of freeing in a sense. It was fearful and scary—it wasn't without all that—but I really enjoyed being with other women and listening to their stories and trying to identify where they were coming from because I do really well with that. If I hear other people sharing their experiences, that helps me to get my stuff out."

> "I think the fact that I could actually share with other women my pain, where I came from because I was always minimizing it or trying to forgive people from the past, trying to let it go, trying—you know. So this way, in the group, I find, I found that other women could share their stories, and I could be free to do it too."

2. The second theme that emerged in the interviews was participants' reflections on how the group helped them challenge and relearn their relational patterns and schemas and enabled them to rebuild their relational capacities. The group and the techniques employed in the group, particularly its focus on affective connection, enabled them to be more emotionally connected, which extended to their experiences outside the group as well, serving as an "ecological bridge" (Mendelsohn et al., 2007). The group helped members consider how to disclose information about themselves and explore the validity of their interpersonal perceptions. Participants highlighted the value of having group members and leaders respond differently than did the people in their past—and being open to taking in this new feedback. This new perspective helped participants realize that they could modulate their sharing and modeled a stance of self-compassion. For example:

"I might just have emotions, but it was hard for me to sit with them. I could name them, but to be actually present to them, then to be present with them in front of another person, was something I wasn't used to. So, I needed some space to be slowed down enough in order to actually be present with them. And then have other people respond in ways that were different from the past so that I could actually encounter and take in new information about how people might react to where I'm at. And so it was just gaining new experiences was what I was looking for."

"I'm working in the group really hard on just accepting my perceptions as being valid, you know. And reflecting on how I want to live my life and not, you know. I'm just trying to get out of the whole black–white, playing games, just the type of way we think about things typically."

"There was one moment where [the group leader] just actually, just kind of, didn't try to move me along but just kind of nodded, gave me a sympathetic look, and I actually took that in. It was like I could feel it at that moment. And that was toward the end of the group, and then she was able to sort of explain what it was. And when she did that it helped me understand—it was what I was wanting, was witnessing, which isn't what I experienced at all in my own trauma history. So, I think there was a way in which—it's not that I needed other people to validate what I needed, but somehow having an experience of that allowed me to hold it a little bit more. And then that very week when I was at home by myself, I was having an emotional flashback—like I was just . . . I could feel fear just building up, and I knew it wasn't in response to any of my current circumstances. All I did was call up a friend of mine and what I asked her to do was "You don't need to say anything, I just need to know you are present. All I just need to know is that someone's there." And then she didn't say a word, and then through that process, as I started talking to myself, I actually had, for the first time, a moment where I actually felt self-compassion, which was huge for me."

One group member reflected on how the group enabled her to better understand her own impact on others because she had struggled to feel a sense of self or sense of self-integrity. Another member reflected on interpersonal conflict that arose in the group which was painful because it mirrored issues from her past but also helped her work through the experience in the group and reassess her ability to cope:

"The way I think about it now is that gave me the opportunity to look at some things that I never would have looked at. It gave me the opportunity to work through a really difficult situation which in past times in group settings like that I would have just left. I wouldn't have gone back, because I experienced it as painful, as a rejection, as a sort of reiteration of what my mother had said. . . . In general, I think it is positive in that I was able to work through that. I was able to go back to the group and finish it, whereas before I would have just left. And I also got the opportunity to think about situations in which people believe or don't believe me and what my reaction is to that and how I could better cope with that. And my therapist said something that really made sense to me and said it was 3 days of a meltdown, whereas a year ago I might have had 3 weeks or 3 months. So, in that regard, I am stronger than I was before. So, I am coping better than I was before. And this was good that it let me see that I can cope."

3. Participants in the group also reflected on how the group enabled them to work on understanding the more subtle aspects of trauma and how it affected their lives. This new perception was an especially relevant issue because the group is designed for members who have typically done a significant amount of work on reducing their trauma symptoms and are hoping to address more complex and unyielding problems in their experience of themselves and their relationships.

One participant spoke about how she was able to integrate further her childhood trauma experiences into her larger life history, which is one of the general goals of the group:

"One of the things that happened that was helpful, I think, is that I was asked to think about the impact of how I grew up and how that either affected my behavior or led me down a path, which is something I was very resistant to do before. I felt like I was being disloyal to my family, but I don't feel so much that way any more. It helped me get a different sort of handle on it and integrate my childhood and other parts of my life, you know. Because there was never a smoking gun for me, so it was really hard to say that this particular thing caused this. It was more just probably my parents and I were not a good fit, you know. And styles of dealing with life—and it was hard on me, and it was hard on them too, I think. But it helped me really integrate that part of my life into the whole history."

Other members also spoke to how the experience in group therapy gave them a new perspective on their family of origin. For example:

"Before—like I said—I was always trying to minimize or I was the problem or I was at fault. Now it is like maybe I wasn't getting what I needed in that family. I wasn't nurtured. I was more of an object, I believe. I think that is what shifted in my therapy and the group. I found out that I was more than an object. One woman said to me, 'it sounds like John Ramsey', when I kind of . . . And I thought, wow, because I was adopted and just for show, just for . . . It was always about the outside with my parents, what the family was going to think about, what the neighbors were going to . . . And it wasn't really about what mattered about me. So, I think, I think just little bits and pieces . . . Realistically I have looked and seen this, you know."

4. Finally, participants also referred to more symptomatic or concrete changes that occurred over the course of the therapy. These changes included being more alert, having a better memory of day-to-day things, feeling more integrated, being better equipped at seeing when emotions are being triggered and also perseverating less over emotional triggers. They referred to an increased capacity to tolerate negative emotions and being able to feel a broader range of emotions, including anger. Participants also noted an improvement in impulsive and anxious behavior. These results correspond well with the changes identified in the self-report data, particularly improvements regarding depression, PTSD, dissociation, and affect regulation. Participants also noted that being in a group of this kind helped them become more focused on the changes they were working toward in their lives in general. For example:

"I felt like I dealt long ago with the depression, but [I'm dealing] more recently with shoplifting and thinking that maybe that is not a good thing to do. So, I have been able to refrain from that, and I think that is because of the group and because of listening to other people talk about how they struggle with that. I am better able to check in with myself, and when I have to urge to [shoplift] I realize that it is when I feel very deprived and powerless, and that is just not an appropriate way to assert power, and it would have disastrous consequences if I did that and were caught. So, I have been able to [end it,] and that is a huge shift since the group."

"I had been biting my nails all through my life as a nervous anxiety thing, I guess. And I wore fake nails for over 20 years, covering up my bitten nails. And for some reason, through the group, I was able to take those nails off and grow my own nails."

"I think participating in the group helped me narrow my original goal and helped me focus more on getting myself out of that housing and understand more of why I feel the way I do about working in certain environments. And that was a huge piece of why I feel like I am unemployable."

Discussion

The TRG is a unique group model for many reasons, but especially so because an important source of healing in the group is identified as the compassionate and validating interactions of group members. The combined outcome data illustrate that, as hypothesized, we observed symptomatic improvements and increased capacity for affect regulation in both the self-report and qualitative data. Further, a decrease in interpersonal problems and conflicts was reflected in both sets of data. In the interview data, we were able to obtain a more in-depth look at how these issues were affected by group treatment. Participants reflected on how the group experience enabled them to challenge and relearn their relational patterns, which then extended to their outside lives. As noted above, tolerating conflict and associated negative affect sufficiently to remain engaged with the group and ultimately enable a resolution was a key aspect of one member's recovery experience. Several participants referenced the power of having group members and co-leaders respond differently to them than the people in their past as fundamental in challenging interpersonal schemas that were no longer adaptive.

As has been noted, impaired self-reference is a particularly pernicious effect of prolonged interpersonal violence. Improvement in self-esteem over the course of this group was a prominent finding in the self-report data. The narrative data permitted one to have a closer and more complex look at the nature of these changes. The interview material illuminated the ways in which the group created an environment in which members discovered that they are capable of both giving and receiving compassion. Client narratives spoke to their experiences of acceptance, belonging, and mutuality in the group. This experience of care and compassion for and from the group appears to have translated into greater self-care and acceptance. As observed earlier, the acceptance of other group members is a powerful antidote to feelings of shame and self-blame. Therefore, although a change in dysfunctional core beliefs about self did not emerge as a significant finding in the self-report data, it may be the case that this concept is more difficult to capture quantitatively and narrative interviews may be better suited to elucidating more textured changes.

Finally, the qualitative data were able to capture some of the more complex and subtle aspects of trauma integration that can occur with this group model that are difficult to assess by using self-report methods. For example, part of the theoretical framework for this group suggests that this modality may be useful for people who have done some work on their trauma histories but want to pursue a goal in an area of their lives in which they feel "stuck," or overwhelmed. The support of the group can be crucial in enabling them to do so, and clients spoke to this issue in their interviews.

CONCLUSION

In summary, the data we have collected in the VOV Program by using quantitative symptom, self-esteem, affect regulation, and relational measures provides a larger-scale naturalistic perspective on gains made in TRG therapy as applied to a diverse and multiply traumatized population. This perspective is complemented by the data from qualitative interviews, which provide a new level of depth and nuance to our understanding of what these changes look like for individuals who have participated in the group. These integrated outcome measures shed preliminary but encouraging light on the effectiveness of the TRG in addressing not only symptoms but also the impact of interpersonal trauma on oneself and one's relationships.

Sample Recruitment Flyer for Clients

TRAUMA RECOVERY GROUP

This is a 16-week goal-oriented, professionally co-led group focusing on decreasing the impact of past trauma on your current life through structured work on a specific aspect of your recovery.

If you are a woman who:

- has been a victim of trauma or abuse
- has done some trauma-focused work in individual therapy
- has achieved some control over posttraumatic symptoms and would like to further understand and decrease the impact of your trauma history on your present life
- has not engaged in self-harming behavior, substance abuse, or been hospitalized during the past year

. . . then this may be the group for you!

Location: _____

Day of week and time: _____

Anticipated starting date: _____

For additional information about joining, please contact: _____

_____

From *The Trauma Recovery Group: A Guide for Practitioners* by Michaela Mendelsohn, Judith Lewis Herman, Emily Schatzow, Melissa Coco, Diya Kallivayalil, and Jocelyn Levitan. Copyright 2011 by The Guilford Press. Permission to photocopy this appendix is granted to purchasers of this book for personal use only (see copyright page for details).

Sample Recruitment Flyer for Clinicians

TRAUMA RECOVERY GROUP

We are currently accepting referrals for a 16-week goal-oriented, professionally co-led group focusing on decreasing the impact of past trauma on current life through structured work on a specific aspect of recovery. Please consider referring women to this group who:

- have been victims or trauma or abuse
- have achieved some control over posttraumatic symptoms and would like to work further on the impact of their trauma history on their present life
- have not engaged in self-harming behavior or substance abuse or been hospitalized for at least the past year
- have done some trauma-focused work in individual therapy

Location: _____

Day of week and time: _____

Anticipated starting date: _____

To make a referral, please contact: _____

_____

From *The Trauma Recovery Group: A Guide for Practitioners* by Michaela Mendelsohn, Judith Lewis Herman, Emily Schatzow, Melissa Coco, Diya Kallivayalil, and Jocelyn Levitan. Copyright 2011 by The Guilford Press. Permission to photocopy this appendix is granted to purchasers of this book for personal use only (see copyright page for details).

APPENDIX C

Telephone Prescreening and Tracking Tool

Hello. I am _____, calling from _____. I am calling in connection with the Trauma Recovery Group. Is this a good time to speak?

First, I want to thank you for your interest and find out a bit about what you are looking for in terms of group treatment. If it seems like this group could be a good match with your needs, I will invite you to come in for an in-person screening interview with me and my co-leader, _____. We will then be able to provide you with further information about the group and discuss whether it may be helpful to you at the present time. If it seems that this group is not a good fit for you, we can make some suggestions about other groups or types of trauma-related work that may be more suitable.

The Trauma Recovery Group is based on the idea that clients at different stages of recovery from trauma have different treatment needs, and the kind of group that is most suitable depends upon where you are in that process. The Trauma Recovery Group is for clients who have done some trauma work in individual and/or group therapy, are currently fairly stable in terms of their symptoms, have developed some positive coping strategies, and do not have any high-risk behaviors. In addition, they have already learned general information about trauma and how it affects them. In this group, clients do a piece of focused work on some aspect of their trauma history and how it is affecting them in the present.

How does this sound so far? [If the potential client is interested, continue. If she is not interested, the conversation can wrap up with appreciation for interest and other referral ideas if possible.]

I would like to ask you a few questions to figure out whether this group might be a good fit with your current treatment needs. I will then speak with the my co-leader and will get back to you within the next few days about whether you should come in for a screening interview or if there is another group that may be more appropriate.

PRESCREENING QUESTIONS

1. How did you hear about this group?
2. Could you please tell me a little about your interest in group treatment at this point?
3. Are you currently in individual therapy? Have you done any work on your trauma history in individual therapy?
4. How are you currently doing with your symptoms? How are you managing in your daily life (e.g., are you working or studying, etc.?)?
5. Within the past year, have you struggled with thoughts of suicide or hurting yourself? Have you acted on any of those thoughts?

(cont.)

From *The Trauma Recovery Group: A Guide for Practitioners* by Michaela Mendelsohn, Judith Lewis Herman, Emily Schatzow, Melissa Coco, Diya Kallivayalil, and Jocelyn Levitan. Copyright 2011 by The Guilford Press. Permission to photocopy this appendix is granted to purchasers of this book for personal use only (see copyright page for details).

6. Have you or anyone else been concerned about your substance use in the past year?
7. Do you currently have any concern about your physical safety?
8. Are you anticipating any major life changes in the next 6 months?
9. Would you be able to attend regular group therapy sessions on [day of week] at [specified time] for an hour and a half between [starting date] and [ending date]?

Thank you very much for speaking with me. I will be back in touch with you as soon as I have had an opportunity to talk with my co-leader about the information that we have discussed. When is the best time to reach you?

TELEPHONE SCREENING TRACKING TOOL

Name: _____

Telephone number(s): _____

Best time to call: _____

Treating clinician and contact number: _____

How heard about group: _____

Prescreening Criteria	Yes	No	Comments
Individual therapy			
Prior trauma work			
Overwhelmed by symptoms			
Suicidal/self-harming behaviors past year			
Substance abuse past year			
Psychiatric hospitalization past year			
Current concerns about physical safety			
Anticipating major life change(s)			
Available for duration of group			

Outcome Tracking:

Screening interview: ____ Yes ____ No

Preferred appointment days/times: _____

Scheduled: _____

Screening Interview Checklist

General client demographics
☐ Age _____   ☐ Ethnic/cultural background _____   ☐ Sexual orientation _____
Overview of current treatments
☐ Individual therapy: nature and duration, trauma focus   ☐ Medications: nature and duration, dosage, effectiveness   ☐ Other treatments
Overview of past treatments and key areas of focus
☐ Individual   ☐ Group   ☐ Others
Interest in pursuing this group therapy at this time
☐ Who initiated the referral?   ☐ Client's hopes, expectations, and concerns

(cont.)

From *The Trauma Recovery Group: A Guide for Practitioners* by Michaela Mendelsohn, Judith Lewis Herman, Emily Schatzow, Melissa Coco, Diya Kallivayalil, and Jocelyn Levitan. Copyright 2011 by The Guilford Press. Permission to photocopy this appendix is granted to purchasers of this book for personal use only (see copyright page for details).

Overview of client's trauma history

□ Nature, duration

□ Who was the perpetrator?

□ Who knew about the abuse? How did he and/or she react or intervene (if at all)?

□ What has the client's experience been as it relates to disclosure?

□ How does the client imagine she will feel when talking about her trauma history in group sessions?

□ How does the client imagine she will feel when hearing about others' traumatic experiences?

Current impact of trauma

□ Symptoms and triggers

□ Impact on day-to-day functioning (work, relationships, etc.)

□ How badly does the client feel when her symptoms are at their worst?

(cont.)

Assessment of coping skills

☐ How does the client manage symptoms?

☐ What kinds of supports (interpersonal, spiritual) does she have available?

☐ What would she do if symptoms were temporarily worsened by the group therapy?

Assessment of risk factors/potential rule-outs

☐ Recent suicidal or self-harming behavior: nature, approximate dates, triggers

☐ Recent psychiatric hospitalization: nature, approximate dates, reasons

☐ Current or recent psychosis

☐ Substance use: nature, quantity, and frequency; history of problems; current supports for sobriety

☐ Current safeguards against violence: any ongoing abuse or close contact with the perpetrator?

☐ Any current or anticipated major life events?

Preliminary goal ideas

☐ Possible goals

☐ Relevance to trauma history and current life

☐ Is it possible to foresee a way in which the goal can be operationalized?

Commitment to attending group

☐ Can the client commit to punctuality and regular attendance?

☐ Does the client anticipate any absences?

Guide for Collateral Contact with the Client's Individual Therapist

Group member: _____

Therapist/Contact name: _____

Phone number: _____

PREGROUP CONTACT WITH INDIVIDUAL THERAPIST

1. Inform the therapist of the group structure, goal focus, and the role of individual therapy in supporting the client's TRG goal work and processing the group experience.
2. Does the therapist think this group is a good match for this client?
3. Does the therapist have any concerns about the client's participation? Does she feel the client would use her individual therapist to address issues that arise from group participation?
4. Share the client's goal ideas. Does the therapist concur with these or have other suggestions?
5. Ask questions eliciting specific information about the client that you need to have clarified (e.g., her particular strengths, safety concerns, her inclination to follow through, nature of between-session contacts).
6. "Is there any additional information that you would like to share?"
7. Inform the therapist about the anticipated time line for decision making and the group anticipated starting date, and provide him or her with contact information for both co-leaders.

MIDGROUP CONTACT WITH INDIVIDUAL THERAPIST

1. Communicate the client's progress toward achieving her goals and her attitudes in participating in the group.
2. Elicit the therapist's feedback and discuss any concerns.
3. "To what extent are TRG material and dynamics being addressed and processed in individual therapy?"
4. If invited, offer suggestions for how the individual therapist might further facilitate the client's better use of TRG therapy.

(cont.)

From *The Trauma Recovery Group: A Guide for Practitioners* by Michaela Mendelsohn, Judith Lewis Herman, Emily Schatzow, Melissa Coco, Diya Kallivayalil, and Jocelyn Levitan. Copyright 2011 by The Guilford Press. Permission to photocopy this appendix is granted to purchasers of this book for personal use only (see copyright page for details).

CONTACT WITH INDIVIDUAL THERAPIST AT THE CONCLUSION OF TRG THERAPY

1. Summarize the client's progress in regard to her goals.
2. Share your recommendations for "next steps."
3. Invite feedback from individual therapist about the client's experience of TRG therapy.

ADDITIONAL CONTACTS WITH THE INDIVIDUAL THERAPIST

1. Date and reason for the contact.
2. Summarize the content.
3. What was the outcome?

Trauma Recovery Group Guidelines

Group time and day: _____

Starting/End dates: _____

Co-leader contact information: _____

_____

Group guidelines are designed to promote feelings of safety and predictability within the group. Please feel free to ask any questions related to these expectations as they occur to you. This handout is a summary of what we have discussed together.

Confidentiality. All information shared in the group must remain confidential (with the exception of conversations held within the context of your individual therapy). If you are seeking the support of friends or family members regarding the group, please be sure to discuss only information relevant to you and to leave out or disguise specific details regarding other members.

Mutual respect. It is important that members interact respectfully by listening to and not interrupting one another. Respect also includes honoring one another's experiences—even when they are hard to understand—and mindfulness regarding others' needs and requests relating to feedback. Thoughtfully asked questions are often a way of expressing respect. Disagreement is acceptable and can be helpful when expressed in a respectful way. "I" statements often help with this process.

No out-of-group contact. Interactions outside of the group session should be limited to pleasantries and should never include information relevant to the group. Options for continued contact after the therapy is completed will be discussed as the end date for the group approaches.

No touching of others. Please remember to use words instead to convey whatever you may feel moved to express through touch. For many trauma survivors, touch can seem very unsafe.

No food. While it is acceptable to bring nonalcoholic beverages to sessions, food can be distracting and is therefore not allowed in sessions.

Lateness and absences. Please make every effort to arrive on time. If you are going to be late for any reason, please inform the group co-leaders ahead of time preferably or as soon as possible. Report any anticipated absences as early as possible to both group co-leaders so that other members can be informed of the reason for your absence in advance.

From *The Trauma Recovery Group: A Guide for Practitioners* by Michaela Mendelsohn, Judith Lewis Herman, Emily Schatzow, Melissa Coco, Diya Kallivayalil, and Jocelyn Levitan. Copyright 2011 by The Guilford Press. Permission to photocopy this appendix is granted to purchasers of this book for personal use only (see copyright page for details).

Co-leader's Group Tracking Notes for Supervisory Meetings

Date: _____

Session number _____ of _____

Who took goal-work time during this group session?

Summarize the goal work and the feedback for each member who used time during this session. Pay close attention to goal development and the content of the feedback and its source.

What interpersonal dynamics are evolving and/or are foreseeable in this group?

(cont.)

From *The Trauma Recovery Group: A Guide for Practitioners* by Michaela Mendelsohn, Judith Lewis Herman, Emily Schatzow, Melissa Coco, Diya Kallivayalil, and Jocelyn Levitan. Copyright 2011 by The Guilford Press. Permission to photocopy this appendix is granted to purchasers of this book for personal use only (see copyright page for details).

What specific group concerns or questions need to be discussed in supervisory meetings?

Which members are taking goal-work time during the next session? What are the related questions or concerns?

What co-leadership considerations or difficulties need to be discussed in supervisory meetings?

Time-Taking Tracking Tool

Co-leaders complete this form outside of group time following Session 1 or 2 (and later on, as needed) when the order of participants' turn taking has been established. Cycle through the order repeatedly, with three clients taking time each week. If the group has fewer or more than six members, the use of this tool is especially important in eliminating confusion or error. It is also helpful in monitoring changes (e.g., if the cycle is disrupted by a group member's absence) and in keeping track of how many "turns" a client has left before the end of the therapy.

Week _____

   Member _____

   Member _____

   Member _____

Week _____

   Member _____

   Member _____

   Member _____

Week _____

   Member _____

   Member _____

   Member _____

Week _____

   Member _____

   Member _____

   Member _____

Week _____

   Member _____

   Member _____

   Member _____

Week _____

   Member _____

   Member _____

   Member _____

Week _____

   Member _____

   Member _____

   Member _____

Week _____

   Member _____

   Member _____

   Member _____

. . . Repeat rotation through the concluding phase.

From *The Trauma Recovery Group: A Guide for Practitioners* by Michaela Mendelsohn, Judith Lewis Herman, Emily Schatzow, Melissa Coco, Diya Kallivayalil, and Jocelyn Levitan. Copyright 2011 by The Guilford Press. Permission to photocopy this appendix is granted to purchasers of this book for personal use only (see copyright page for details).

Member's Concluding Exercise Preparation

SELF-ASSESSMENT

1. What was my goal?

2. What did I accomplish in relation to my original goal?

3. What might be a possible next step I will take as a result of being in this group?

4. What imaginary gift will I give to myself related to my work in this group?

PEER FEEDBACK

Consider the same questions as they relate to each other member of the group: Use this as a tool to remind you of thoughts you would like to share. Please remember to protect group member confidentiality in your note writing.

Member 1:

Member 2:

(cont.)

From *The Trauma Recovery Group: A Guide for Practitioners* by Michaela Mendelsohn, Judith Lewis Herman, Emily Schatzow, Melissa Coco, Diya Kallivayalil, and Jocelyn Levitan. Copyright 2011 by The Guilford Press. Permission to photocopy this appendix is granted to purchasers of this book for personal use only (see copyright page for details).

Member 3:

Member 4:

Member 5:

CO-LEADER AND GROUP FEEDBACK

1. What did you like most about the group?

2. What did you like least about the group?

3. What did the co-leaders do that was helpful?

4. What should the co-leaders do differently in future groups?

5. Do you have any other feedback about the group experience?

APPENDIX J

Supervisor's Tracking Tool

Member's name: _____

Relevant history:

Goal tracking (including process of operationalizing goal and any changes during group sessions):

trauma-related ____   present-oriented ____   achievable ____   concrete ____   specific ____

(cont.)

From *The Trauma Recovery Group: A Guide for Practitioners* by Michaela Mendelsohn, Judith Lewis Herman, Emily Schatzow, Melissa Coco, Diya Kallivayalil, and Jocelyn Levitan. Copyright 2011 by The Guilford Press. Permission to photocopy this appendix is granted to purchasers of this book for personal use only (see copyright page for details).

Participation (sharing/feedback, etc.):

Concluding session feedback:

References

Alexander, P. C., Neimeyer, R. A., Follette, V. M., Moore, M. K., & Harter, S. (1989). A comparison of group treatments of women sexually abused as children. *Journal of Consulting and Clinical Psychology, 57,* 479–483.

Allen, S. N., & Bloom, S. L. (1994). Group and family treatment of post-traumatic stress disorder. *Psychiatric Clinics of North America, 17,* 425–437.

American Psychiatric Association. (1994). *Diagnostic and statistical manual of mental disorders* (4th ed.). Washington, DC: Author.

Arata, C. M., Langhinrichsen-Rohling, J., Bowers, D., & O'Farrill-Swails, L. (2005). Single versus multi-type maltreatment: An examination of the long-term effects of child abuse. *Journal of Aggression, Maltreatment, and Trauma, 11,* 29–52.

Barkham, M., Hardy, G. E., & Startup, M. (1996). The IIP-32: A short version of the Inventory of Interpersonal Problems. *British Journal of Clinical Psychology, 35,* 21–35.

Beck, A. T., Ward, C. H., Mendelson, M., Mock, J., & Erbaugh, J. (1961). An inventory for measuring depression. *Archives of General Psychiatry, 4,* 561–571.

Beck, A. T., Steer, R. A., & Garbin, M. G. (1988). Psychometric properties of the Beck Depression Inventory: Twenty-five years of evaluation. *Clinical Psychology Review, 8,* 77–100.

Benedek, D. M., Friedman, M. J., Zatzick, D., & Ursano, R. J. (2009). Guideline watch (March 2009): Practice guideline for the treatment of patients with acute stress disorder and posttraumatic stress disorder. *Focus, 7,* 204–213.

Bernard, H. S., & Mackenzie, K. R. (Eds.). (1994). *Basics of group psychotherapy.* New York: Guilford Press.

Bernstein, E. M., & Putnam, F. W. (1986). Development, reliability, and validity of a dissociation scale. *Journal of Nervous and Mental Disease, 174,* 727–735.

Blascovich, J., & Tomaka, J. (1991). Measures of self-esteem. In J. P. Robinson, P. R. Shaver, & L. S. Wrightsman (Eds.), *Measures of personality and social psychological attitudes* (Vol. I, pp. 115–160). San Diego, CA: Academic Press.

Boston Globe Investigative Staff. (2002). *Betrayal: The crisis in the Catholic Church.* Boston: Little, Brown.

Boudewyn, A. C., & Liem, J. H. (1995). Childhood sexual abuse as a precursor to depression and self-destructive behavior in adulthood. *Journal of Traumatic Stress, 8,* 445–459.

Bradley, R., Greene, J., Russ, E., Dutra, L., & Westen, D. (2005). A multidimensional meta-analysis of psychotherapy for PTSD. *American Journal of Psychiatry, 162,* 214–227.

Bradley, R. G., & Follingstad, D. R. (2003). Group therapy for incarcerated women who experienced interpersonal violence: A pilot study. *Journal of Traumatic Stress, 16,* 337–340.

Briere, J. (1996). *Therapy for adults molested as children* (2nd ed., exp. and rev.). New York: Springer.

Briere, J., & Jordan, C. E. (2004). Violence against women: Outcome complexity and implications for assessment and treatment. *Journal of Interpersonal Violence, 19,* 1252–1276.

Briere, J., & Jordan, C. E. (2009). The relationship between childhood maltreatment, moderating variable, and adult psychological difficulties in women: An overview. *Trauma, Violence and Abuse: A Review Journal, 10,* 375–388.

Briere, J., & Rickards, S. (2007). Self-awareness, affect regulation, and relatedness: Differential sequels of childhood versus adult victimization experiences. *Journal of Nervous and Mental Disease, 195,* 497–503.

Briere, J., & Runtz, M. (1993). Childhood sexual abuse: Long-term sequelae and implications for psychological assessment. *Journal of Interpersonal Violence, 8,* 312–330.

Briere, J., & Scott, C. (2006). *Principles of trauma therapy: A guide to symptoms, evaluation, and treatment.* Thousand Oaks, CA: Sage.

Brom, D., Kleber, R. J., & Defares, P. B. (1989). Brief psychotherapy for posttraumatic stress disorders. *Journal of Consulting and Clinical Psychology, 57,* 607–612.

Browne, A., & Bassuk, S. S. (1997). Intimate violence in the lives of homeless and poor housed women: Prevalence and patterns in an ethnically diverse sample. *American Journal of Orthopsychiatry, 67,* 261–278.

Browne, A., Miller, B., & Maguin, E. (1999). Prevalence and severity of lifetime physical and sexual victimization among incarcerated women. *International Journal of Law and Psychiatry, 22,* 301–322.

Bryer, J. B., Nelson, B. A., Miller, J. D., & Krol, P. A. (1987). Childhood physical and sexual abuse as factors in adult psychiatric illness. *American Journal of Psychiatry, 144,* 1426–1430.

Carlson, E. B., & Putnam, F. W. (1993). An update on the Dissociative Experiences Scale. *Dissociation, 6,* 16–27.

Chard, K. M. (2005). An evaluation of Cognitive Processing Therapy for the treatment of posttraumatic stress disorder related to childhood sexual abuse. *Journal of Consulting and Clinical Psychology, 73,* 965–971.

Charuvastra, A., & Cloitre, M. (2008). Social bonds and posttraumatic stress disorder. *Annual Review of Psychology, 59,* 301–328.

Chu, J. A. (1988). Ten traps for therapists in the treatment of trauma survivors. *Dissociation, 1,* 24–32.

Chu, J. A., & Dill, D. L. (1990). Dissociative symptoms in relation to childhood physical and sexual abuse. *American Journal of Psychiatry, 147,* 887–892.

Classen, C. C., Koopman, C., Nevill-Manning, K., & Speigel, D. (2001). A preliminary report comparing trauma-focused and present-focused group therapy against a wait-listed control condition among childhood sexual abuse survivors with PTSD. *Journal of Aggression, Maltreatment and Trauma, 4,* 265–288.

Classen, C. C., Palesh, O. G., & Aggarwal, R. (2005). Sexual revictimization: A review of the empirical literature. *Trauma, Violence, and Abuse, 6,* 103–129.

Cloitre, M., Cohen, L. R., & Koenen, K. C. (2006). *Treating survivors of childhood abuse: Psychotherapy for the interrupted life.* New York: Guilford Press.

Cloitre, M., Koenen, K. C., Cohen, L. R., & Han, H. (2002). Skills training in affective and interpersonal regulation followed by exposure: A phase-based treatment for PTSD related to childhood abuse. *Journal of Consulting and Clinical Psychology, 70,* 1067–1074.

Cloitre, M., Miranda, R., Stovall-McClough, C., & Han, H. (2005). Beyond PTSD: Emotion regulation and interpersonal problems as predictors of functional impairment in survivors of childhood abuse. *Behavior Therapy, 36,* 199–124.

Cohen, L. R., Hien, D. A., & Batchelder, S. (2008). The impact of cumulative maternal trauma and diagnosis on parenting behavior. *Child Maltreatment, 13,* 27–38.

Coid, J., Petrukevitch, A., Feder, G., Chung, S., Richardson, J., & Moorey, S. (2001). Relation between childhood sexual and physical abuse and risk of revictimization in women: A cross-sectional study. *The Lancet, 358,* 450–454.

Convention on the Elimination of All Forms of Discrimination against Women. (1979). Retrieved on September 9, 2010, from *www.un.org/womenwatch/daw/cedaw.*

Cook, J. M., Schnurr, P. P., & Foa, E. B. (2004). Bridging the gap between posttraumatic stress disorder research and clinical practice: The example of exposure therapy. *Psychotherapy: Theory, Research, Practice, Training, 41,* 374–387.

Cook, T. D., & Campbell, D. T. (1979). *Quasi-experimentation: Design and analysis for field settings.* Chicago: Rand McNally.

Courtois, C. (1997). Treating the sexual concerns of adult incest survivors and their partners. *Journal of Aggression, Maltreatment and Trauma, 1,* 293–310.

Courtois, C. A., & Ford, J. D. (Eds.). (2009). *Treating complex traumatic stress disorders: An evidence-based guide.* New York: Guilford Press.

Courtois, C. A., Ford, J. D., & Cloitre, M. (2009). Best practices in psychotherapy for adults. In C. A. Courtois & J. D. Ford (Eds.), *Treating complex traumatic stress disorders: An evidence-based guide* (pp. 82–103). New York: Guilford Press.

Creswell, J. W. (1998). *Qualitative inquiry and research design: Choosing among the five traditions.* Thousand Oaks, CA: Sage.

Daigneault, I., Cyr, M., & Tourigny, M. (2007). Exploration of recovery trajectories in sexually abused adolescents. *Journal of Aggression, Maltreatment and Trauma, 14,* 165–184.

David, D., Giron, A., & Mellman, T. A. (1995). Panic–phobic patients and developmental trauma. *Journal of Clinical Psychology, 56,* 113–117.

Davidson, P. R., & Parker, K. C. (2001). Eye movement desensitization and reprocessing (EMDR): A meta-analysis. *Journal of Consulting and Clinical Psychology, 69,* 305–316.

de Groot, J. M., & Rodin, G. M. (1999). The relationship between eating disorders and childhood trauma. *Psychiatric Annals, 29,* 225–229.

Delucia-Waack, J. L., & Fauth, J. (2004). Effective supervision of group leaders: Current theory, research and implications for practice. In J. L. Delucia-Waack, D. A. Gerrity, C. R. Kalodner, & M. T. Riva (Eds.), *Handbook of group counseling and psychotherapy* (pp. 136–151). Thousand Oaks, CA: Sage.

Delucia-Waack, J. L., Gerrity, D. A., Kalodner, C. R., & Riva, M. T. (Eds.). (2004). *Handbook of group counseling and psychotherapy.* Thousand Oaks, CA: Sage.

Denzin, N. K., & Lincoln, Y. S. (1998). Entering the field of qualitative research. In N. K. Denzin & Y. S. Lincoln (Eds.), *Strategies of qualitative inquiry* (pp. 1–35). London: Sage.

Desai, R. A., Harpaz-Rotem, I., Najavits, L. M., & Rosenheck, R. A. (2008). Impact of seeking safety program on clinical outcomes among homeless female veterans with psychiatric disorders. *Psychiatric Services, 59,* 996–1003.

Dube, S. R., Anda, R. F., Felitti, V. J., Chapman, D. P., Williamson, D. F., & Giles, W. H. (2001). Childhood abuse, household dysfunction, and the risk of attempted suicide throughout the lifespan: Findings from the Adverse Childhood Experiences study. *Journal of the American Medical Association, 286,* 3089–3096.

Dube, S. R., Anda, R. F., Whitfield, C. L., Brown, D. W., Felitti, V. J., Dong, M., et al. (2005). Long-term consequences of childhood sexual abuse by gender of victim. *American Journal of Preventive Medicine, 28,* 430–438.

Dube, S. R., Felitti, V. J., Dong, M., Chapman, D. P., Giles, W. H., & Anda, R. E. (2003). Childhood abuse, neglect, and household dysfunction and the risk of illicit drug use: The adverse childhood experiences study. *Pediatrics, 111*, 564–572.

Edwards, V. J., Holden, G. W., Felitti, V. J., & Anda, R. F. (2003). Relationship between multiple forms of childhood maltreatment and adult mental health in community respondents: Results from the Adverse Childhood Experiences study. *American Journal of Psychiatry, 160*, 1453–1460.

Erturk, Y. (2009, June). *Fifteen Years of the United Nations Special Rapporteur on Violence against Women, its Causes and Consequences (1994–2009): A Critical Review.* United Nations Human Rights Council, 11th session.

Farley, M. (2008, June 20). U.N. deems sexual attacks a security issue. *Los Angeles Times.* Retrieved February 2, 2010, from *articles.latimes.com/2008/jun/20/world/fg-violence20.*

Finzi-Dottan, R., & Karu, T. (2006). From emotional abuse in childhood to psychopathology in adulthood: A path mediated by immature defense mechanisms and self-esteem. *Journal of Nervous and Mental Disease, 194*, 616–621.

Foa, E. B. (1997). Trauma and women: Course, predictors, and treatment. *Journal of Clinical Psychiatry, 58*, 25–28.

Foa, E. B., Cashman, L., Jaycox, L., & Perry, K. (1997). The validation of a self-report measure of posttraumatic stress disorder: The Posttraumatic Diagnostic Scale. *Psychological Assessment, 9*, 445–451.

Foa, E. B., Keane, T. M., & Friedman, M. J. (Eds.). (2000). *Effective treatment for PTSD: Practice guidelines from the International Society for Traumatic Stress Studies.* New York: Guilford Press.

Foa, E. B., & Rothbaum, B. O. (1998). *Treating the trauma of rape: Cognitive behavioral therapy for PTSD.* New York: Guilford Press.

Fonagy, P., Target, M., Gergely, G., Allen, J. G., & Bateman, A. W. (2003). The developmental roots of borderline personality disorder in early attachment relationships: A theory and some evidence. *Psychoanalytic Inquiry, 23*, 412–459.

Ford, J. D., & Courtois, C. A. (2009). Defining and understanding complex trauma and complex traumatic stress disorders. In C. A. Courtois & J. D. Ford (Eds.), *Treating complex traumatic stress disorders: An evidence-based guide* (pp. 13–30). New York: Guilford Press.

Ford, J. D., Courtois, C. A., Steele, K., van der Hart, O., & Nijenhuis, E. R. S. (2005). Treatment of complex posttraumatic self-dysregulation. *Journal of Traumatic Stress, 18*, 437–447.

Fosha, D. (2000). *The transforming power of affect: A model of accelerated change.* New York: Basic Books.

Foy, D. W., Glynn, S. M., Schnurr, P. P., Jankowski, M. K., Wattenberg, M. S., Weiss, D. S., et al. (2000). Group therapy. In E. B. Foa, T. M. Keane, & M. J. Friedman (Eds.), *Effective treatments for PTSD* (pp. 155–175). New York: Guilford Press.

Foy, D. W., Schnurr, P. P., Weiss, D. S., Wattenberg, M. S., Glynn, S. M., Marmar, C. R., et al. (2001). Group psychotherapy for PTSD. In J. P. Wilson, M. J. Friedman, & J. D. Lindy (Eds.), *Treating psychological trauma and PTSD* (pp. 183–202). New York: Guilford Press.

Fritch, A. M., & Lynch, S. M. (2008). Group treatment for adult survivors of interpersonal trauma. *Journal of Psychological Trauma, 7*, 145–169.

Gillock, K. L., Zayfert, C., Hegel, M. T., & Ferguson, R. J. (2005). Posttraumatic stress disorder in primary care: Prevalence and relationships with physical symptoms and medical utilization. *General Hospital Psychiatry, 27*, 392–399.

Gratz, K. L., & Roemer, L. (2004). Multidimensional assessment of emotion regulation and dysregulation: Development, factor structure, and initial validation of the Difficulties in Emotion Regulation Scale. *Journal of Psychopathology and Behavioral Assessment, 26*, 41–54.

Harney, P. A., & Harvey, M. R. (1999). Group psychotherapy: An overview. In B. H. Young & D. D.

Blake (Eds.), *Group treatments for post-traumatic stress disorder* (pp. 1–13). New York: Brunner/Mazel.

Harris, M. (1998). *T.R.E.M. Trauma Recovery and Empowerment: A clinician's guide to working with women in groups.* New York: Free Press.

Harvey, M. R. (1996). An ecological view of psychological trauma and trauma recovery. *Journal of Traumatic Stress, 9,* 3–23.

Harvey, M. R., & Tummala-Narra, P. (Eds.). (2007). *Sources and expressions of resiliency in trauma survivors: Ecological theory, multicultural practice.* Binghamton, NY: Haworth Maltreatment & Trauma Press.

Harvey, M. R., Westen, D., Lebowitz, L., Saunders, E., Avi-Yonah, O., & Harney, P. (1994). *Multidimensional Trauma Recovery and Resiliency Interview (MTRR-I).* Unpublished manuscript, Victims of Violence Program, Department of Psychiatry, Cambridge Health Alliance, Cambridge, MA.

Hazzard, A., Rogers, J. H., & Angert, L. (1993). Factors affecting group therapy outcome for adult sexual abuse survivors. *International Journal of Group Psychotherapy, 43,* 453–468.

Herman, J., & Schatzow, E. (1984). Time-limited group therapy for women with a history of incest. *International Journal of Group Psychotherapy, 34,* 605–615.

Herman, J. L. (1986). Histories of violence in an outpatient population. *American Journal of Orthopsychiatry, 56,* 137–141.

Herman, J. L. (1988). Considering sex offenders: A model of addiction. *Signs: Journal of Women in Culture and Society, 13,* 695–724.

Herman, J. L. (1992a). Complex PTSD: A syndrome in survivors of prolonged and repeated trauma. *Journal of Traumatic Stress, 3,* 377–391.

Herman, J. L. (1992b). *Trauma and recovery.* New York: Basic Books.

Herman, J. L., & Hirschman, L (1977). Father–daughter incest. *Signs: Journal of Women in Culture and Society, 2,* 735–756.

Herman, J. L., Perry J. C., & van der Kolk, B. A. (1989). Childhood trauma in borderline personality disorder. *American Journal of Psychiatry, 146,* 490–495.

Herman, J. L., Russell, D. E. H., & Trocki, K. (1986). Long-term effects of incestuous abuse in childhood. *American Journal of Psychiatry, 143,* 1293–1296.

Hien, D., & Scheier, J. (1996). Trauma and short-term outcome for women in detoxification. *Journal of Substance Abuse Treatment, 13,* 227–231.

Hien, D. A., Cohen, L. R., Miele, G. M., Litt, L. C., & Capstick, C. (2004). Promising treatments for women with comorbid PTSD and substance use disorders. *American Journal of Psychiatry, 161,* 1426–1432.

Holmes, W. C., & Slap, G. B. (1998). Sexual abuse of boys: Definition, prevalence, correlates, sequelae, and management. *Journal of the American Medical Association, 280,* 1855–1162.

Horowitz, L., Rosenberg, S. E., Baer, B. A., Ureno, G., & Villasenor, V. S. (1988). Inventory of Interpersonal Problems: Psychometric Properties and Clinical Applications. *Journal of Consulting and Clinical Psychology, 56,* 885–892.

Horowitz, M. J. (1997). *Stress response syndromes* (3rd ed.). Northvale, NJ: Aronson.

House, A. S. (2006). Increasing the usability of Cognitive Processing Therapy for survivors of child sexual abuse. *Journal of Child Sexual Abuse, 15,* 87–103.

Izutsu, T., Shibuya, M., Tsutsumi, A., Konishi, T., & Kawamura, N. (2008). The relationship between past traumatic experiences and sickness absence. *International Journal of Social Psychiatry, 54,* 83–89.

Jacobson, A. (1989). Physical and sexual assault histories among psychiatric outpatients. *American Journal of Psychiatry, 146,* 755–758.

Jacobson, A., & Richardson, B. (1987). Assault experiences of 100 psychiatric inpatients: Evidence of the need for routine inquiry. *American Journal of Psychiatry, 144,* 980–913.

Janoff-Bulman, R. (1992). *Shattered Assumptions: Towards a New Psychology of Trauma.* New York: Free Press.

Journal of Traumatic Stress. (2005). Special section on complex trauma, *18*(5).

Kaplan, H., & Sadock, B. (Eds.). (1994). *Comprehensive group psychotherapy.* Baltimore, MD: Williams & Wilkins.

Keane, T. M., Marshall, A. D., & Taft, C. T. (2006). Posttraumatic stress disorder: Etiology, epidemiology, and treatment outcome. *Annual Review of Clinical Psychology, 2,* 161–197.

Kessler, R. C., Sonnega, A., Bromet, E., Hughes, M., & Nelson, C. B. (1995). Posttraumatic stress disorder in the National Comorbidity Survey. *Archive of General Psychiatry, 52,* 1048–1060.

Kilpatrick, D. G., Veronen, L. J., & Resick, P. A. (1982). Psychological sequelae to rape: Assessment and treatment strategies. In D. M. Doleys, R. I. Meredity, & A. R. Ciminero (Eds.), *Behavioral medicine: Assessment and treatment strategies* (pp. 473—497). New York: Plenum Press.

Kimerling, R., Gima, K., Smith, M. W., Street, A., & Frayne, S. (2007). The Veterans Health Administration and military sexual trauma. *American Journal of Public Health, 97*(12), 2160–2166.

Kimerling, R. E., Alvarez, J., Pavao, J. R., Mack, K. P., Smith, M. W., & Baumrind, N. (2009). Unemployment among women: Examining the relationship of physical and psychological intimate partner violence and posttraumatic stress disorder. *Journal of Interpersonal Violence, 24,* 450–463.

Klein, R. H., & Schermer, V. L. (Eds.). (2000). *Group psychotherapy for psychological trauma.* New York: Guilford Press.

Korn, D. L., & Leeds, A. M. (2002). Preliminary evidence of efficacy for EMDR resource development and installation in the stabilization phase of treatment of complex posttraumatic stress disorder. *Journal of Clinical Psychology, 58,* 1465–1487.

Koss, M. P., Bailey, J. A., & Yuan, N. P. (2003). Depression and PTSD in survivors of male violence: Research and training initiatives to facilitate recovery. *Psychology of Women Quarterly, 27,* 130–142.

Koss, M. P., & Harvey, M. A. (1991). *The rape victim: Clinical and community interventions* (2nd ed.). Thousand Oaks, CA: Sage.

Krippner, S., & McIntyre, T. M. (Eds.). (2003). *Psychological impact of war trauma on civilians: An international perspective.* Santa Barbara, CA: Greenwood.

Krupnick, J. L. (2002). Brief psychodynamic treatment of PTSD. *Journal of Clinical Psychology/In Session: Psychotherapy in Practice, 58,* 919–932.

Lansen, J., & Haans, T. (2004). Clinical supervision for trauma therapists. In J. P. Wilson & B. Drozdek (Eds.), *Broken spirits: The treatment of traumatized asylum seekers, refugees, war and torture victims* (pp. 317–354). New York: Brunner-Routledge.

Lauterbach, D., Bak, C., Reiland, S., Mason, S., Lute, M. R., & Earls, L. (2007). Quality of parental relationships among persons with a lifetime history of posttraumatic stress disorder. *Journal of Traumatic Stress, 20,* 161–172.

Lebowitz, L., Harvey, M. R., & Herman, J. L. (1993). A stage-by-dimension model of recovery from sexual trauma. *Journal of Interpersonal Violence, 8,* 378–391.

Leserman, J. (2005). Sexual abuse history: Prevalence, health effects, mediators, and psychological treatments. *Psychosomatic Medicine, 67,* 906–915.

Lifton, R. J. (1973). *Home from the war: Vietnam veterans: Neither victims nor executioners.* New York: Simon & Schuster.

Lubin, H., & Johnson, D. R. (2008). *Trauma-centered group psychotherapy for women: A clinician's manual.* Philadelphia, PA: Haworth Press.

Lubin, H., Loris, M., Burt, J., & Johnson, D. R. (1998). Efficacy of psychoeducational group therapy in reducing symptoms of posttraumatic stress disorder among multiply traumatized women. *American Journal of Psychiatry, 155,* 1172–1177.

Mann, J. (1973). *Time-limited psychotherapy.* Cambridge, MA: Harvard University Press.

Mann, J. (1996). Time-limited psychotherapy. In J. E. Groves (Ed.), *Essential papers on short-term dynamic therapy* (pp. 66–96). New York: NYU Press. (Original work published 1973)

Marin, A. J., & Russo, N. P. (1999). Feminist perspectives on male violence again women: Critiquing O'Neil and Harway's model. In M. Harway & J. M. O'Neil (Eds.), *What causes men's violence against women?* (pp. 18–35). Thousand Oaks, CA: Sage.

McCann, I. L., & Pearlman, L. A. (1990). Vicarious traumatization: A framework for understanding the psychological effects of working with victims. *Journal of Traumatic Stress, 3*, 131–149.

McCauley, J., Kern, D. E., Kolodner, K., Dill, L., Schroeder, A. F., DeChant, H. K., et al. (1995). The "battering syndrome": Prevalence and clinical characteristics of domestic violence in primary care internal medicine practices. *Annals of Internal Medicine, 123*, 737–746.

McHugo, G. J., Caspi, Y., Kammerer, N., Mazelis, R., Jackson, E. W., Russell, L., et al. (2005). The assessment of trauma history in women with co-occurring substance abuse and mental disorders and a history of interpersonal violence. *Journal of Behavioral Health Services and Research, 32*, 113–127.

Mendelsohn, M., Zachary, R., & Harney, P. (2007). Group therapy as an ecological bridge to a new community. *Journal of Aggression, Maltreatment and Trauma, 14*, 227–243.

Miller, J. B. (1976). *Towards a new psychology of women*. Boston: Beacon Press.

Miller, J. B. (1990). *Connections, disconnections, and violations* (Work in Progress No. 33). Wellesley, MA: Stone Center, Working Paper Series.

Mitchell, J. (1966). The longest revolution, *New Left Review, 40*, 11–37.

Mitchell, J. (1971). *Women's estate*. New York: Pantheon.

Mishler, E. G. (2004). Historians of the self: Restorying lives, revising identities. *Research in Human Development, 1*, 103–123.

Morgan, T., & Cummings, A. L. (1999). Change experienced during group therapy by female survivors of child sexual abuse. *Journal of Consulting and Clinical Psychology, 67*, 28–36.

Mueser, K. T., Salyers, M. P., Rosenberg, S. D., Goodman, L. A., Essock, S. M., Osher, F. C., et al. (2004). Interpersonal trauma and posttraumatic stress disorder in patients with severe mental illness: Demographic, clinical and health correlates. *Schizophrenia Bulletin, 30*, 45–57.

Najavits, L. M. (2002). *Seeking Safety: A treatment manual for PTSD and substance abuse*. New York: Guilford Press.

Najavits, L. M., Weiss, R. D., & Shaw, S. R. (1997). The link between substance abuse and posttraumatic stress disorder in women: A research review. *American Journal on Addictions, 6*, 273–283.

Najavits, L. M., Weiss, R. D., Shaw, S. R., & Muenz, L. R. (1998). "Seeking safety": Outcome of a new cognitive-behavioral psychotherapy for women with posttraumatic stress disorder and substance dependence. *Journal of Traumatic Stress, 11*, 437–456.

Nemeroff, C. B., Bremner, D., Foa, E. B., Mayberg, H. S., North, C. S., & Stein, M. B. (2006). Posttraumatic stress disorder: A state-of the-science review. *Journal of Psychiatric Research, 40*, 1–21.

Neria, Y., Olfson, M., Gameroff, M. J., Wickramaratne, P., Pilowsky, D., Verdeli, H., et al. (2008). Trauma exposure and posttraumatic stress disorder among primary care patients with bipolar spectrum disorder. *Bipolar Disorders, 10*, 503–510.

Noll, J. G., Trickett, P. K., Harris, W. W., & Putnam, F. W. (2009). The cumulative burden borne by offspring whose mothers were sexually abused as children: Descriptive results from a multigenerational study. *Journal of Interpersonal Violence, 24*, 424–449.

Ogata, S. N., Silk, K. R., & Goodrich, S. (1990). Childhood sexual and physical abuse in adult patients with borderline personality disorder. *American Journal of Psychiatry, 147*, 1008–1013.

Ogden, P., Minton, K., & Pain, C. (2006). *Trauma and the body: A sensorimotor approach to psychotherapy*. New York: Norton.

Osterman, J. E., & de Jong, J. T. V. M. (2007). Cultural issues and trauma. In M. J. Friedman, T. M.

Keane, & P. A. Resick (Eds.), *Handbook of PTSD: Science and practice* (pp. 425–447). New York: Guilford Press.

Pearlman, L. A., & Courtois, C. A. (2005). Clinical applications of the attachment framework: Relational treatment of complex trauma. *Journal of Traumatic Stress, 18*, 449–460.

Peddle, N. (2007). Assessing trauma impact, recovery, and resiliency in refugees of war. *Journal of Aggression, Maltreatment and Trauma, 14*, 185–204.

Putnam, F. W., Guroff, J. J., Silberman, E. K., Barban, L., & Post, R. M. (1986). The clinical phenomenology of multiple personality disorder: Review of 100 recent cases. *Journal of Clinical Psychology, 47*, 285–293.

Reinharz, S. T. (1992). *Feminist methods in social research.* London: Oxford University Press.

Rennie, D. L., Phillips, J. R., & Quartaro, G. K. (1988). Grounded theory: A promising approach to conceptualization in psychology? *Canadian Psychology, 29*, 139–150.

Resick, P. A. (2001). Cognitive therapy for posttraumatic stress disorder. *Journal of Cognitive Psychotherapy, 15*, 321–330.

Resick, P. A., Monson, C. M., & Gutner, C. (2007). Psychosocial treatments for PTSD. In M. J. Friedman, T. M. Keane, & P. A. Resick (Eds.), *Handbook of PTSD: Science and practice* (pp. 330–358). New York: Guilford Press.

Resick, P. A., Nishith, P., Weaver, T. L., Astin, M. C., & Feuer, C. A. (2002). A comparison of cognitive-processing therapy with prolonged exposure and a waiting condition for the treatment of chronic posttraumatic stress disorder in female rape victims. *Journal of Consulting and Clinical Psychology, 70*, 867–879.

Resick, P. A., & Schnicke, M. K. (1993). *Cognitive processing therapy for rape victims: A treatment manual.* Newbury Park, CA: Sage.

Rich, C. L., Combs-Lane, A. M., Resnick, H. S., & Kilpatrick, D. G. (2004). Child sexual abuse and adult sexual revictimization. In L. J. Koenig, L. S., Doll, A. O'Leary, & W. Pequegnat (Eds.), *From child sexual abuse to adult sexual risk: Trauma, revictimization, and intervention* (pp. 49–68). Washington, DC: American Psychological Association.

Richter, N. L., Snider, E., & Gorey, K. M. (1997). Group work intervention with female survivors of childhood sexual abuse. *Research on Social Work Practice, 7*, 53–69.

Roelofs, K., Keijsers, G. P. J., Hoogduin, K. A. L., Näring, G. W. B., & Moene, F. C. (2002). Childhood abuse in patients with conversion disorder. *American Journal of Psychiatry, 159*, 1908–1913.

Romans, S. E., Belaise, C., Martin, J. L., Morris, E., & Raffi, A. (2002). Childhood abuse and later medical disorders in women: An epidemiological study. *Psychotherapy and Psychosomatics, 71*, 141–150.

Rosenberg, M. (1965). *Society and the adolescent self-image.* Princeton, NJ: Princeton University Press.

Rosenthal, L. (2005). Group supervision of groups: A modern analytic perspective. *Modern Psychoanalysis, 30*, 167–184.

Rothbaum, B. O., Meadows, E. A., Resick, P., & Foy, D. W. (2000). Cognitive-behavioral therapy. In E. B. Foa, T. M. Keane, & M. J. Friedman (Eds.), *Effective treatments for PTSD* (pp. 60–83). New York: Guilford Press.

Rutan, J. S., Stone, W. N., & Shay, J. J. (2007). *Psychodynamic group psychotherapy* (4th ed.). New York: Guilford Press.

Ryan, M., Nitsun, M., Gilbert, L., & Mason, H. (2005). A prospective study of the effectiveness of group and individual psychotherapy for women CSA survivors. *Psychology and Psychotherapy: Theory, Research and Practice, 78*, 465–479.

Salston, M., & Figley, C. R. (2003). Secondary traumatic stress effects of working with survivors of criminal victimization. *Journal of Traumatic Stress, 16*, 167–174.

Sarwer, D. B., & Durlak, J. A. (1996). Childhood sexual abuse as a predictor of adult female sexual dysfunction: A study of couples seeking sex therapy. *Child Abuse and Neglect, 20*, 963–972.

Schatzow, E., & Herman, J. L. (1989). Breaking secrecy: Adult survivors disclose to their families. *Psychiatric Clinics of North America, 12*(2), 337–349.

Schmitt, D. P., & Allik, J. (2005). Exploring the universal and culture-specific features of global self-esteem. *Journal of Personality and Social Psychology, 89*, 623–642.

Schottenbauer, M. A., Glass, C. R., Arnkoff, D. B., & Gray, S. H. (2008). Contributions of psychodynamic approaches to treatment of PTSD and trauma: A review of the empirical treatment and psychopathology literature. *Psychiatry, 71*, 13–34.

Schottenbauer, M. A., Glass, C. R., Arnkoff, D. B., Tendick, V., & Gray, S. H. (2008). Nonresponse and dropout rates in outcome studies on PTSD: Review and methodological considerations. *Psychiatry, 71*, 134–168.

Schwartz, R. C. (1995). *Internal family systems therapy.* New York: Guilford Press.

Seligman, M. E. P. (1972). Learned helplessness. *Annual Review of Medicine, 23*, 407–412.

Shapiro, F. (1989). Efficacy of eye movement desensitization procedure in the treatment of traumatic memories. *Journal of Traumatic Stress, 2*, 199–223.

Skinner, K. M., Kressin, N., Frayne, S., Tripp, T. J., Hankin, C. S., Miller, D. R., et al. (2000). The prevalence of military sexual trauma among female Veterans' Administration outpatients. *Journal of Interpersonal Violence, 15*, 291–310.

Solomon, S. D., & Johnson, D. M. (2002). Psychosocial treatment of posttraumatic stress disorder: A practice-friendly review of outcome research. *Journal of Clinical Psychology/In Session: Psychotherapy in Practice, 58*, 947–959.

Spinazzola, J., Blaustein, M., & van der Kolk, B. A. (2005). Posttraumatic stress disorder treatment outcome research: The study of unrepresentative samples? *Journal of Traumatic Stress, 18*, 425–436.

Stein, M. B., Lang, A. J., Laffaye, C., Satz, L. E., Lenox, R. J., & Dresselhaus, T. R. (2004). Relationship of sexual assault history to somatic symptoms and health anxiety in women. *General Hospital Psychiatry, 26*, 178–183.

Stein, M. B., McQuaid, J. R., Pedrelli, P., Lenox, R., & McCahill, M. E. (2000). Posttraumatic stress disorder in the primary care medical setting. *General Hospital Psychiatry, 22*, 261–269.

Strauss, A., & Corbin, J. (1990). *Basics of qualitative research: Grounded theory procedures and techniques.* Newbury Park, CA: Sage.

Surrey, J., Stiver, I. P., Miller, J. B., Kaplan, A., & Jordan, J. V. (1991). *Women's growth in connection: Writings from the Stone Center.* Wellesley, MA: Wellesley Center for Women.

Switzer, G. E., Dew, M. A., Thompson, K., Goycoolea, J. M., Derricott, T., & Mullins, S. D. (1999). Posttraumatic stress disorder and service utilization among urban mental health center clients. *Journal of Traumatic Stress, 12*, 25–39.

Thompson, M. P., Kaslow, N. J., Kingree, J. B., Puett, R., Thompson, N. J., & Meadows, L. (1999). Partner abuse and posttraumatic stress disorder as risk factors for suicide attempts in a sample of low-income, inner-city women. *Journal of Traumatic Stress, 12*, 59–72.

Tjaden, P., & Thoennes, N. (2000). *Full report of the prevalence, incidence and consequences of violence against women: Findings from the National Violence Against Women Survey* (NCJ 183781). Washington, DC: U.S. Department of Justice.

Toussaint, D. W., VanDeMark, N. R., Bornemann, A., & Graeber, C. J. (2007). Modifications to the Trauma Recovery and Empowerment Model (TREM) for substance-abusing women with histories of violence: Outcomes and lessons learned at a Colorado substance abuse treatment center. *Journal of Community Psychology, 35*, 879–894.

Tucker, P., & Trautman, R. (2000). Understanding and treating PTSD: Past, present, and future. *Bulletin of the Menninger Clinic, 64*, A37–A51.

Tummala-Narra, P. (2007). Conceptualizing trauma and resilience across diverse contexts: A multicultural perspective. *Journal of Aggression, Maltreatment and Trauma, 14*, 33–54.

Tummala-Narra, P., Liang, B., & Harvey, M. R. (2007). Aspects of safe attachment in the recovery from trauma. *Journal of Aggression, Maltreatment and Trauma, 14*(3), 1–18.

Twombly, J. H. (2000). Incorporating EMDR and EMDR adaptations into the treatment of clients with dissociate identity disorder. *Journal of Trauma and Dissociation, 1*, 61–81.

United Nations General Assembly. (1993). *Declaration on the Elimination of Violence against Women.* G.A. Res. 48/104, 48 U.N. GAOR Supp. (No. 49) at 217, U.N. Doc. A/48/49.

United Nations Population Fund. (2000, October). *Lives together, worlds apart: Men and women in a time of change.* New York: United Nations Population Fund.

van der Kolk, B. A. (1996). The complexity of adaptation to trauma: Self-regulation, stimulus discrimination, and characterological development. In B. A. van der Kolk, A. C. McFarlane, & L. Weisaeth (Eds.), *Traumatic stress: The effects of overwhelming experience on mind, body, and society* (pp. 182–213). New York: Guilford Press.

van der Kolk, B. A., Pelcovitz, D., Roth, S., Mandel, F., McFarlane, A., & Herman J. L. (1996). Dissociation, affect dysregulation and somatization: The complexity of adaptation to trauma. *American Journal of Psychiatry, 153*(Festschrift Suppl.), 83–93.

van der Kolk, B. A., Perry, J. C., & Herman, J. L. (1991). Childhood origins of self-destructive behavior. *American Journal of Psychiatry, 148*, 1665–1671.

van der Kolk, B. A., Roth, S., Pelcovitz, D., Sunday, S., & Spinazzola, J. (2005). Disorders of extreme stress: The empirical foundation of a complex adaptation to trauma. *Journal of Traumatic Stress, 18*, 389–399.

Van IJzendoorn, M. H., & Schuengel, C. (1996). The measurement of dissociation in normal and clinical populations: Meta-analytic validation of the Dissociative Experiences Scale (DES). *Clinical Psychology Review, 16*, 365–382.

Walker, E. A., Gelfand, A. N., Katon, W. J., Koss, M. P., Von Korff, M., Bernstein, D., et al. (1999). Adult health status of women with histories of childhood abuse and neglect. *American Journal of Medicine, 107*, 332–339.

Walker, L. (2000). *The battered woman syndrome* (2nd ed.). New York: Springer.

Walker, M. (2004). Supervising practitioners working with survivors of childhood abuse: Countertransference, secondary traumatization and terror. *Psychodynamic Practice, 10*, 173–193.

Weathers, F. W., Litz, B. T., & Keane, T. M. (1995). Military trauma. In J. R. Freedy & S. E. Hobfoll (Eds.), *Traumatic stress: From theory to practice* (pp. 103–128). New York: Plenum Press.

Weeks, R., & Widom, C. S. (1998). Self-reports of early childhood victimization among incarcerated adult male felons. *Journal of Interpersonal Violence, 13*, 346–361.

Welburn, K., Coristine, M., Dagg, P., Pontefract, A., & Jordan, S. (2002). The Schema Questionnaire-Short Form: Factor Analysis and Relationship between Schemas and Symptoms. *Cognitive Therapy and Research, 26*, 519–530.

Westbury, E., & Tutty, L. M. (1999). The efficacy of group treatment for survivors of childhood abuse. *Child Abuse and Neglect, 23*, 31–44.

Westen, D., Ludolph, P., & Misle, B. (1990). Physical and sexual abuse in adolescent girls with borderline personality disorder. *American Journal of Orthopsychiatry, 60*, 55–66.

Whetten, K., Leserman, J., Lowe, K., Stangl, D., Thielman, N., Swartz, M., et al. (2006). Prevalence of childhood sexual abuse and physical trauma in an HIV-positive sample from the Deep South. *American Journal of Public Health, 96*, 1028–1030.

Wilson, J. P., Friedman, M. J., & Lindy, J. D. (Eds.). (2001). *Treating psychological trauma and PTSD.* New York: Guilford Press.

Wolfsdorf, B. L., & Zlotnick, C. (2001). Affect-management group for survivors of sexual abuse. *Journal of Clinical Psychology/In Session: Psychotherapy in Practice, 57*, 169–182.

Wonderlich, S. A., Crosby, R. D., Mitchell, J. E., Thompson, K. M., Redlin, J., Demuth, G., et al. (2001). Eating disturbance and sexual trauma in childhood and adulthood. *International Journal of Eating Disorders, 30,* 401–412.

Yalom, I. D., & Leszcz, M. (2005). *The theory and practice of group psychotherapy* (5th ed.). New York: Perseus Books.

Young, B. H., & Blake, D. D. (Eds.). (1999). *Group treatments for post-traumatic stress disorder.* New York: Brunner/Mazel.

Young, J. E., & Brown, G. (2003). *Young Schema Questionnaire: Short Form.* New York: Cognitive Therapy Center of New York.

Zinzow, H. M., Grubaugh, A. L., Monnier, J., Suffoletta-Maierle, S., & Frueh, B. C. (2007). Trauma among female veterans: A critical review. *Trauma, Violence and Abuse, 8,* 384–400.

Zlotnick, C., Shea, M. T., Rosen, K. H., Simpson, E., Mulrenin, K., Begin, A., et al. (1997). An affect-management group for women with posttraumatic stress disorder and histories of childhood sexual abuse. *Journal of Traumatic Stress, 10,* 425–436.

Zlotnick, C., Johnson, J. E., Kohn, R., Vicente, B., Rioseco, P., & Saldivia, S. (2008). Childhood trauma, trauma in adulthood, and psychiatric diagnoses: Results from a community sample. *Comprehensive Psychiatry, 49,* 163–169.

Zoellner, L. A., Fitzgibbons, L. A., & Foa, E. B. (2001). Cognitive-behavioral approaches to PTSD. In J. P. Wilson, M. J. Friedman, & J. D. Lindy (Eds.), *Treating psychological trauma and PTSD* (pp. 159–182). New York: Guilford Press.

Zugazaga, C. (2004). Stressful life event experiences of homeless adults: A comparison of single men, single women, and women with children. *Journal of Community Psychology, 32,* 643–654.

Index